HORSEFEATHERS

HORSEFEATHERS

FACTS VERSUS MYTHS ABOUT YOUR HORSE'S HEALTH

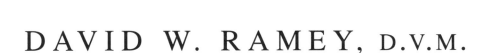

DAVID W. RAMEY, D.V.M.

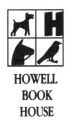

HOWELL
BOOK
HOUSE

NEW YORK

The information contained in this book is not intended as a substitute for the advice of a veterinarian. The reader is advised to consult a veterinarian in all matters relating to a horse's health.

HOWELL BOOK HOUSE
A Prentice Hall Macmillan Company
15 Columbus Circle
New York, NY 10023

MACMILLAN is a registered trademark of Macmillan, Inc.

Library of Congress Cataloging-in-Publication Data

Ramey, David W.
    Horsefeathers : facts versus myths about your horse's health /
David W. Ramey.
        p. cm.
    Includes bibliographical references and index.
    ISBN 0–87605–986–8
    1. Horses—Health. 2. Horses—Diseases. I. Title.
SF951.R24 1995
636.1'089—dc20   94–24195
                    CIP

Manufactured in the United States of America
10 9 8 7 6 5 4 3 2 1

Truth lies somewhere if we knew but where

WILLIAM COWPER

Contents

Preface   ix
Acknowledgments   xii

PART I: THE THINGS DONE TO (AND FOR) HORSES

1. Diagnostics	3
2. Therapeutics	18
3. Drugs	32

PART II: FEEDS AND FEEDING

4. What's in the Feed?	49
5. Feeding the Adult Horse	54
6. Youth, Pregnancy and Other Stresses	65

PART III: ROUTINE CARE

7. Vaccinations	75
8. Deworming	88
9. Teeth	96

PART IV: WHEN THINGS GO WRONG

10. Colics	105
11. Strangles	116
12. Wounds	122

PART V: *THE MUSCULOSKELETAL SYSTEM*

13. Legs	135
14. Hooves	151
15. Navicular Disease (The Big Myth)	165

PART VI: *MISCELLANY*

16. Behavior	179
17. Pet Peeves	188

Epilogue   193
Notes   195
Index   209

Preface

Horses have an inexplicable grip on those who love and care for them. The author, an equine veterinarian, was not raised around horses. Rather, on his first serious exposure to them he was stricken with the equine bug. This has led to daily dealings with horses and their owners, an experience that has limitless rewards, fascinations and frustrations.

Foremost among the frustrations are the huge number of stories about how horses are "supposed" to be taken care of. Most of this dogma is based on experiences and anecdotes of undoubtedly well-meaning and sincere horse owners, trainers, feed store owners and even veterinarians. Unfortunately, these are often backed with limited expertise or mistaken beliefs. For well-meaning horse owners, these axioms, tales and myths present a formidable obstacle to the goal of being comfortable with their favorite animal's health.

All of what people do to and for horses is done with the horse's "best" interests in mind. What is best for the horse, of course, depends on whom you ask. Most people do things with pure motives; they want to help and do good. The fact that someone is unqualified to render an opinion rarely overrides this impulse to try and help.

Opinions are like belly buttons; everyone has one. However, not all opinions should be given equal weight. When searching for help, the horse owner should make some attempt to seek out a qualified opinion. Experience, though a good teacher, is not a substitute for study and training. Accordingly, there is a terrific amount of bad information, gained purely by "experience," that is spread around liberally by horse "experts." For horse owners, this bewildering mass of information merely adds to the confusion about what to do for their horses.

As anyone with parents knows, having someone make all of your decisions for you is not always in your own best interest. Invariably your parents just didn't "understand" the situation. Horses, of course, find themselves in the same position as you did with your parents. Understanding horse health is particularly difficult because all of the information about them is based on observations of how the horses respond to whatever it is that is done to them. You can't, after all, ask the horse how he's doing (with apologies to psychic enthusiasts). You must do what you think is best and then watch and see what happens.

This being said, it is important to keep in mind a simple principle of logic. Just because *b* follows *a* doesn't mean that *a* caused *b*. For example, assume that your horse is limping *(b)*. Then also say that the farrier changed your horse's shoes yesterday *(a)*. The two may be related. But they may not. Your horse could have kicked something in the stall and hurt his foot. It is far too easy (and tempting) to give the credit or the blame to the obvious. You certainly don't want to ignore the obvious possibility that the horse was shod improperly. At the same time, you don't want to overlook something else.

Say, for example, your horse seems a bit off. You give him his favorite treat: warm bran and carrots. Several hours later you conclude that he's better. Was it because of the bran and carrots? Could it have been the few hours (time heals all wounds)? Could you have been wrong in the first place (the horse was really okay)? Is the horse learning that if he acts in a certain way he's going to get a treat? An open mind is a quality to cherish and an essential component of drawing reasonable conclusions.

Horses have virtually no input into the decisions that are made for them. They are surprisingly amenable to being fussed over (being tolerant creatures that generally bite and kick only when pressed). The best thing that the poor horse can hope for is that his owner will be sensible in what he or she expects, take care of any problems that come up and feed him regularly. He is likely to put up with incessant brushing, continuous hoof polishing, wild costuming, trailering, showing and a variety of other ailments as long as he gets treated reasonably well. Horses did quite well as a species prior to man's figuring out that they would put up with a rider. Much of what is said to be necessary placates the owner more than it helps the horse.

In some ways, horses are like cars. You have a car. What does it need? Regular maintenance, gas and oil are about the only essentials. Some of you, however, use a pine-scented air freshener, have fuzzy dice on the rear-view mirror and have chrome wheel covers. While these are (debatably) wonderful, they are by no means necessary for the good health of your car.

Horses are kind of like that, too. As long as you take care of a few basic things, everything will most likely be just fine. Just like your car, they may have the occasional breakdown, but the majority of them are repairable.

Finally, you, as a horse owner, have to be reasonable. There are not reasons or answers for every problem. Working on horses is a challenging undertaking, at best. Horses don't like to undergo the poking and prodding that is required for even the most basic examinations. They are unable to voice what their problems are and probably wouldn't if they could. They are notoriously bad patients who refuse to take care of themselves and view any attempt at rest or confinement as a terrible imposition on their desires to run and play. They often seem to try *not* to get better.

Have some compassion for the people who are trying to help you with your uncooperative and ungrateful beast and let them do the best they can at trying to help. Nobody has all the answers. People who are willing to tell you that they don't know are at least telling you the truth.

It is for the entertainment, enlightenment, information and soothing of the poor, distressed horse owner that this manual of equine mythology is designed. This book takes on a huge variety of misconceptions about the health of the horse and attempts to point the reader in the direction of the truth. Because some of these myths are firmly held, the book is referenced, both for credibility and to help the reader find additional information. The author knows that facts frequently have no chance at dislodging firmly held misconceptions but feels that at least they are worth taking a shot at. This is not a comprehensive book on horse health, but rather an attempt to shed some light on problems facing the horse owner, trainer and veterinarian. With any luck, horses will benefit, too.

Acknowledgments

No book can be completed without help. I could not have finished this work without the proofreading and suggestions of the "beautiful and brilliant" Patricia Friedland. Madelyn Larsen, the editor, was patient, thoughtful and encouraging from the moment I started. It was my good fortune to receive my veterinary education at Colorado State University, where a practical approach to problems was encouraged, and to matriculate under the eye of Dr. Eric Reinertson, at Iowa State University, who let me explore. To my clients, from whom all of my source material came, I owe thanks for my veterinary practice and for their concern for the welfare of their friends. Finally, to Mary French, patient and intelligent proofreader, olive goddess, yeoman operator of the copy machine and special friend, thank you for the light.

PART I

THE THINGS DONE TO (AND FOR) HORSES

1

Diagnostics

Being a veterinarian for horses is sort of like being a pediatrician. Generally, your patients don't like you very much, love to be difficult and misbehave and don't like to take their medicine. They are uncooperative and hard to communicate with. Horses are a diagnostic challenge.

People frequently ask, "Isn't it too bad that horses can't talk?" Well, yes and no. On the one hand, it would be nice if horses could be a little bit helpful in describing their symptoms and source of pain or trouble. Conversely, since they can't talk, they can't, for instance, complain or whine about the size of the needle that's coming at them. (They don't ever pass out on seeing needles, either.)

Since horses can't talk, a diagnostician (whoever that may be) must make a careful assessment of the horse's condition, gather data, estimate the response that the horse has to certain stimuli and come up with some sort of rational approach to solving the horse's problem. Diagnostics, even in the best of circumstances (such as at human hospitals), is not always a clear-cut process. The making of a diagnosis is something of a process of trial and error. You make an observation and you try to explain it by gathering data. When the difficulties inherent in working on horses, such as size, strength and obstinacy, are combined with the fact that horses can't tell you what's happening to them (at least not directly) and the fact that medicine is an inexact science, you have a process that is fraught with opportunities for mistakes. Making a diagnosis is something that has to be done carefully. Anyone who tells you quickly and assuredly what the problem is with a horse without bothering to make a thorough examination should be looked at with suspicion.

For example, suppose your friend says, "Your horse looks like he's colicking. Maybe he has a stone."

Well, maybe he does.

Of course, maybe he has something else.

The point is that this sort of snap judgment is almost never useful, accurate or worthy of consideration. It mostly means that your friend is demonstrating concern in a misguided fashion. Whether the friend is right or wrong becomes purely a matter of chance and not something that you should rely on as a basis for treatment.

You, of course, care only that your horse gets better as soon as possible. You want perfection, accuracy and speed of diagnosis, at a reasonable price. While this is certainly desirable, it is also impossible, especially if these goals are demanded every time. The quick stall-side diagnosis made by concerned observers does satisfy a couple of the desired requirements of a "good" diagnosis: it is generally cheap and quick. Unfortunately, the fact that such diagnoses are often inaccurate does not seem to do anything to limit their availability or acceptance. Diagnosis is often a difficult, frustrating and unsatisfying process.

One other thing that must be understood about making a diagnosis is that sometimes even with the best of attention and intentions, a veterinarian can't make one. In human medicine, even with all the equipment and tests available to medical doctors (and patients that talk), sometimes a precise diagnosis cannot be made. This is unfortunate but true. And it will most likely always be the case in both human and veterinary medicine. The best thing that you can hope for in your diagnostician is that he or she is thorough, educated, up to date and professional. Even with those qualities, you can't have perfection in diagnostics, at least not yet. Knowing this, ideally, you will give your veterinarian a break from time to time.

SICK HORSES

The most common sign of a sick horse is that he doesn't seem normal. While this seems terribly obvious, it is also terribly important. Horses are creatures of habit (as are their owners). They tend to act predictably as individuals; that is, horses will tend to act in certain ways all the time. This predictability becomes part of what you like about your horse. You spend a lot of time with your horse, and naturally you will get to know his behavior well.

For instance, say you go to the stall and lovingly call, "Widowmaker." Widowmaker jumps to the front of the stall, straining the stall guard and gnashing his teeth, and pins his ears back. You know that he's fine because this happens every day.

When you see that your horse is sick, you will notice that something has changed in his appearance or his demeanor. The change may be subtle. Widowmaker may not pin his ears back upon hearing his name and may actually let you pet him. Or a change may be obvious, as with a runny nose.

When you call your veterinarian, realize that you know a lot about how your horse acts normally: much more than he or she does. Convey this information. A horse can appear different from normal to you and still seem all right to someone else who is looking at him for the first time. You should try to tell your veterinarian exactly what it is about the way your horse is behaving that you feel is abnormal. This will help get the diagnostic process off to a good

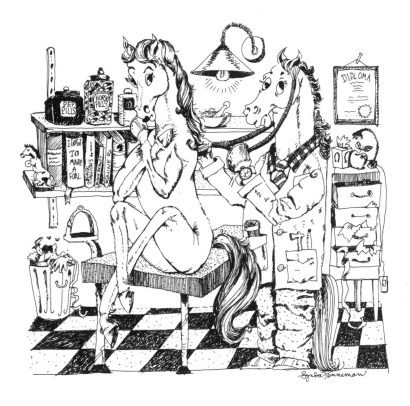

Diagnostics are best left to trained examiners.

start. Then your veterinarian will use one of a number of methods to try to figure out what, if anything, is wrong.

MONITORING BODY SOUNDS

A stethoscope is always useful in making a diagnosis on a sick horse and is a requirement for any veterinarian. If you have a stethoscope, it will make you look very knowledgeable around the barn, even if you don't know how to use it. Using a stethoscope isn't difficult. You put it on and listen to what's going on inside the horse. The tricky part is in knowing how to interpret what you hear.

The horse's body is made up of two big cavities filled with stuff. In the chest cavity, the stuff inside is heart and lungs. In the abdomen, the stuff includes intestines, kidneys, spleen, liver, bladder and reproductive organs.

In the chest, a stethoscope helps you listen to the beating of the heart and the pumping of the lungs. The heartbeat of the horse can have a variety of normal sounds and rhythms, but the lungs should always sound clear and never full of wheezes and gurgles. It's all quite musical.

In the abdomen, you can hear that the intestines are moving, or not. It's always nice to hear sounds in the abdominal cavity (borborygmi), but their presence or absence is rarely diagnostic of anything in and of itself. The abdomen can be quite melodic in its own right, and the groans and pops that you normally hear are always at least a good source of amusement. Gut sounds can be affected by a variety of stimuli. Exercise, for example, will slow down or stop sounds in the gut. If there are no sounds in the abdomen, don't automatically assume the worst.

A good diagnostician will use a stethoscope to try to help identify abnormal sounds. Listening with a stethoscope is really quite an art (like any other form of listening). In the airways, the presence of fluid may result in a variety of "wet" sounds. In the abdomen, certain sounds are associated with the presence of gas or sand.[1] In a colicking horse, these sounds may be significant. The sounds heard with a stethoscope are one step toward a diagnosis.

MONITORING BODY TEMPERATURE

A rectal thermometer tells you the temperature of the horse's body. For adult horses, the normal temperature is between 99.5 and 101°F. If you think that your horse is "a bit off," by all means take his temperature. This is easy enough, and it will provide some useful information for your veterinarian when you call. It will also give you something to do until he or she gets there.

Raising the body temperature is something that horses do with ease, apparently at the slightest provocation. In you, a body temperature rise of two degrees will make you feel pretty awful. Horses very commonly have temperature elevations of three or four degrees with even minor illnesses. Don't believe that your horse's problem is serious just because his temperature is 104.5°F (and by all means don't get hysterical). A body temperature elevation may be a sign of big trouble, but it almost always is not.

An increase in body temperature in and of itself is not a problem. "Fever" is not a disease. In fact, fever may be a good thing. Fever occurs in most species of vertebrate animals and is thought by many to be one of the more primitive ways that the body tries to fight off an infection. Researchers think that the body may raise its temperature in an effort to make the living space for bacteria or viruses (i.e., the horse, in this case) less hospitable for their growth and development, since bacteria and viruses may not grow as well if the temperature is turned up. An increase in the horse's body temperature may really just be a natural response to an infection.[2,3,4,5,6,7,8]

It's interesting that the level of a fever apparently has nothing to do with how sick an animal is.[9] That is, a temperature of 104°F isn't any worse (or better) than a temperature of 102°F. Just because your horse's fever is higher than his sick neighbor's doesn't mean that your horse is somehow worse.

Fever can be bad if it's excessive. Most fevers rarely cause an increase in the body temperature of greater than 2.5°C (about 6.6°F). When they do, they result in decreased survival.[3,10] So if your horse has a fever of about 107°F, you probably do need to take some pains to control the fever itself.

Most of the time, however, your frantic efforts at controlling a horse's temperature, while understandable, are not needed. Fans and ice baths and alcohol rubs mostly make you feel better because you're doing something. Unfortunately, these don't get at the source. If you can find out what the cause of the fever is, perhaps you will be able to take care of it.

Medical science is divided on what to do about fevers. Since fever is a natural response that may help control the spread of the infection, some doctors are tempted to leave fever alone and let it run its course. The presence or absence of a fever can be a useful indicator of how the horse is responding to treatment, too.

From one standpoint, however, not treating a fever can be a risky thing to do for a doctor, unless he or she knows the client well. This is because the veterinarian who does not treat a fever may not be living up to the client's expectations. Since most people want something done for their horses' fever, they will be suspicious of anyone who is *supposed* to do something and then doesn't. When suspicion is compounded by peer pressure ("You mean he didn't give him anything for his fever!!!?"), the veterinarian can really find him- or herself out on a limb. The fact that the veterinarian is the most qualified person to make the decision usually doesn't enter into the equation.

But since horses with fevers don't eat, look and feel bad and tear at our hearts, many people prefer to try to give drugs to control the fever. The non-steroidal anti-inflammatory drugs, such as phenylbutazone (bute), are useful for helping to keep a fever down (more on this later). If controlling a fever with drugs were really harmful, this probably would have been noted a long time ago, since it has been done for such a long time.[6]

What does seem to be agreed upon is that you should either control the fever or not. Most physicians (M.D.s) feel that mild fevers are best left alone, while the high ones should be controlled.[7] If you have decided to try to control your horse's fever, you should administer the appropriate drugs regularly, at intervals designed to prevent peaks and valleys in the fever. If you decide not to try to keep the fever down, you should monitor the horse's temperature and look for signs that the horse is getting better. The choice of whether or not to try to control your horse's fever should be made by your veterinarian and most likely, unless the fever is really high (the ones that *need* to be controlled), either decision is the right one.

THE RECTAL EXAMINATION

For many conditions of the horse, a rectal examination is helpful. Your veterinarian can examine the back portion of your horse's abdominal cavity by this method. This really is quite an interesting and enlightening experience (for the vet, anyway) and horses are surprisingly amenable to it.

Your vet can't feel the entire contents of the abdomen during a rectal examination. Nobody's arm is long enough to do that. Some of the pelvis, the bladder, reproductive structures (in females), the back of the left kidney, some intestines and the edge of the spleen: these are all that can be reached from the rear of the horse (literally). It has been estimated that a good rectal examination will allow the examiner to feel, at best, 40 percent of the contents of the abdomen. Don't expect (or believe) that your vet will feel the liver or stomach or pancreas because it can't happen. Rectals are useful examinations for a variety of conditions. They can, unfortunately, miss a lot, and much depends on the skill of the examiner. Still, rectal examination is a fairly basic diagnostic procedure.[11]

EXAMINATION OF THE BLOOD

Examination of the blood is very useful in helping diagnose problems of the sick horse, although most people think that blood can tell them a lot more than it really can.

Blood is made up of two things: cells and the fluids that the cells travel around in. There are two basic color varieties of blood cell: red and white. (Another type of blood cell, the platelet, is important in blood clotting but it will not be discussed here.)

Measuring Red Blood Cells

Red blood cells have one important function. They tote oxygen around to the various cells of the body. Red blood cells are measured in two ways. First, the numbers of cells can be counted (this is usually done with a machine). Second, and more commonly, a measurement called the packed cell volume is made.[12]

The horse *almost never* has any problems with his red blood cells. There is a huge range in the normal levels of red blood cells. The horse stores extra red blood cells in the spleen. He has a tremendous capacity to increase the amount of red blood cells in the circulation at literally a moment's notice by calling on these extra cells. These can be called into action when more oxygen is needed, for instance, during exercise. It is, unfortunately, impossible to measure the blood cells in the spleen. Therefore, a single blood test does not give a very accurate reflection of the actual number of red blood cells in the horse's body.[13,14]

Problems with too many red blood cells are almost unheard of, but everyone gives lots of attention to a lack of red blood cells, which is called anemia. This can be a serious problem when it occurs in sick horses. In anemia, either not enough red cells are being made or a bunch of them have been lost. Red blood cells can be lost, through bleeding, for example. In some chronic diseases, it is possible that not enough red cells are being produced by the horse's body. However, anemia occurs rarely in horses that appear to be otherwise healthy.

In people, as in horses, anemia can occur for a variety of reasons. Often, in people, a deficiency in iron or B vitamins is diagnosed. Both of these substances are needed for red blood cell production (in both species). Humans have to obtain both iron and B vitamins in their diet. Neither substance is in abundance in the "normal" human diet of hamburgers and french fries.

When iron- or B vitamin–deficient anemias occur in people, people take iron supplements or B vitamins. (This sort of treatment logic is inescapable.)

Naturally, it is inevitable that people will want to do the same things for their horses that they would for themselves.

Anemia, when it occurs, makes people feel bad. Lots of horses get treated for "anemia," too. The story usually goes like this:

> OWNER: My horse doesn't have enough energy.
> TRAINER: Let's draw blood. Maybe he's anemic.
> VETERINARIAN: His packed cell volume is a bit low.
> EVERYONE: Let's give him a supplement!

As a result, the horse may or may not feel better, but to everyone's relief, at least some sort of a "diagnosis" of his condition has been made.

This line of diagnosis and treatment is very common in horses, and very misguided. True iron or vitamin deficiency anemias are almost unknown in horses. The example overlooks too many sources of error to be a reasonable line of thought. First, a single packed cell volume test is not a reliable indicator of the actual number of red blood cells present in the horse's body. Second, horses don't get iron or B vitamin deficiencies, especially when they are fed. Horses get lots of iron, other minerals and B vitamins in their diet. Hay and dirt are loaded with the stuff. The horse also manufactures its own B vitamins.

If a horse is getting enough feed to keep from getting skinny, if he's not starving, then he's getting enough to eat to make red blood cells. Even though the entire diagnostic process, as described above, is easy and simple and even logical, it just doesn't jibe with the medical facts. Even if the horse "responds" to vitamin supplements with a "better" blood test, the response may only reflect an otherwise inconsequential difference in a second blood test. Or it may reflect your desire to see your horse getting better.[15]

If your horse lacks energy, give him energy by giving him more feed (more on this later). Vitamins do not provide energy. Vitamin supplements are no solution to a problem that doesn't exist, even if it is commonly diagnosed.

Measuring White Blood Cell Levels

White blood cell levels go up or down, most commonly due to infections by bacteria or viruses. The body responds to infections by producing white blood cells. They are the front-line shock troops that are sent into the battle to fight off an infection. Their measurement can be useful in helping estimate a horse's response to disease. A high level of white blood cells may indicate that the horse is aggressively fighting off an infection. A low level may mean that the cells are being used up faster than they can be produced. Following their levels as a disease progresses can be a good way to follow a response to treatment.[14]

Serum Measurements

The fluid that the blood cells travel around the body in is called the plasma. If some of the protein is taken out of the plasma, the fluid that is left is called serum. Laboratories take measurements on serum because the protein in the plasma gums up the machines that do the measuring.

Serum measurements are really quite useful. They can be made because the blood system is a kind of trash-removal system for the body's metabolic byproducts. The blood visits all the cells in the body, bringing gifts like nutrients and oxygen. The body takes the gifts and dumps garbage back into the blood. Although this would seem to be an unsatisfactory basis for maintaining a relationship, it apparently works out well enough for the body.

Laboratories measure these metabolic byproducts, along with levels of salts, sugars and proteins, so veterinarians can use them to make indirect assessments about some of the body's tissues. Some of the garbage items are specific to certain tissues. Veterinarians can tell how well the liver is working, for example, by looking at serum levels of enzymes that are found only in the liver. If lots of liver cells die, say from disease, lots of liver-specific enzymes are released into the blood. Or you can tell that the kidney is working fine because certain bits of garbage are removed only by the kidney. When the kidneys don't work, the garbage levels go up (sort of like when city sanitation workers go on strike).

While laboratory measurements of the blood are really useful in helping diagnose certain conditions, they are limited nevertheless. A lot of things, like tumors, or colics, or even many infections, cannot be picked up by testing the blood.

You cannot find out "what is lacking" in your horse by taking a blood test, so don't try. Blood tests do not tell you about vitamin or mineral levels. They are not *that* specific. Don't expect too much from blood tests.

MEASURING OTHER FLUIDS

Besides blood, there are other body fluids that can be looked at. There's fluid in the chest around the lungs, fluid in the abdomen around the guts and fluid in the spinal column around the spinal cord. Fluid is everywhere. Each of these fluids can all be looked at in the laboratory. Analysis of the fluid can provide a good reflection of what's happening in these areas, since a disease process may end up dumping cells into these fluids or otherwise changing their composition. Body fluids are generally not difficult (or dangerous) to obtain. Your veterinarian may recommend looking at them (or even suggest other special tests), while trying to figure out what's wrong with your sick horse.

LAME HORSES

If horses aren't sick or cut, they are commonly lame. Veterinarians spend a good part of any day trying to determine why a particular horse is limping. The whole procedure can be a frustrating and tedious affair. Unless the problem is obvious, like a nail sticking out of the bottom of the foot, your veterinarian will most likely want to employ some sort of diagnostic aids to discover the source of your horse's problem.

MANUAL PALPATION

Manual palpation of a limb is certainly the most commonly used method of lameness diagnosis. Palpation simply means "feeling." A good examiner can detect, among other things, swellings where swellings aren't supposed to be, stiff joints, areas of soreness and increases in pulse to the foot. While some of these factors can be recognized easily, the more subtle instances of their occurrence can be easily overinterpreted, especially when the examiner doesn't know what he or she is doing.

"Doc, my horse hurts here!" says the concerned owner, poking anxiously at a spot on the horse's flank. The horse kicks out and lays his ears back with each successive jab.

The horse hates being poked.

Horses are pretty jumpy creatures. They are not particularly stoic about pain and will jump away from stimuli just because they don't like it. Therefore, the casual or careless application of an unpleasant (though not even particularly painful) stimulus can easily be misinterpreted.

Palpation is the cause of more quick misdiagnoses than you can even imagine. For instance, someone squeezes the muscle at the base of the neck, near where it ties into the shoulder, and your horse jumps. Horses can't stand this. Walk down a barn aisle sometime and see how many horses will stand placidly when you squeeze their neck muscles. You will hear, however, that this is a classic sign of sore shoulders, or soreness from improper leg movement, or some other rot. Nothing of the sort! How do you react if someone pinches you in the muscles that run along the top of your shoulder (like Mr. Spock in the old "Star Trek" series)? Does that mean that you have a problem in that area?

Horses are likely to jump if you poke them in the flank or run your fingers along the muscles of the back. These are sensitive areas. Sure, horses with sore backs don't like to have their back muscles pushed on. A lot of normal horses don't like to have their back muscles pushed on, either.

The point is that while palpation is a useful and essential diagnostic tool, it is also open to variations of technique and interpretation. Anyone who casually palpates your horse, squeezes a muscle and pronounces a "cause" for your horse's problem without at least performing a more thorough examination is at best careless and at worst a charlatan. If you don't know how to palpate your horse, don't be sure that the next person who comes along does, either. Without belaboring the point, the person who should be doing the palpation of your horse is your veterinarian.

If you do think that you palpate something abnormal, like a swelling, but you're not sure, look at the other leg. Horses are conveniently made with another leg that is a mirror image of the one that you are examining. If the thing that you are worried about exists on both legs, it's most likely normal for that particular horse.

CHECKING FOR HEAT

Everybody gets all excited about feeling for "heat" in a horse's leg. Inflamed areas *are* measurably warmer than areas that are not inflamed. An inflamed area is warmer than the surrounding tissue because in areas of inflammation the blood vessels are leaky. Fluid and cells can slip through gaps that occur in the blood vessels that open with inflammation. This is a well-demonstrated effect of inflammation, and it also accounts for the swelling that accompanies the heat. (In people, the redness that you also see in an inflamed area is due to the increased number of red blood cells that leak into an inflamed area.)

Heat in tissue has been demonstrated by using a technique known as thermography.[16] Unfortunately for diagnostic purposes, this technique hasn't been as beneficial or as widely used as veterinarians had initially hoped because numerous factors exist that can make getting accurate results from a thermographic examination difficult. In human medicine, thermography is performed in a very controlled situation. Such things as motion and environmental temperature are much trickier to control in a horse in a barn than in a person in a hospital. Although heat can indicate an area of inflammation, the author's experience is that people misjudge their ability to determine that an area is hotter than normal. Thermography has shown that a one-degree rise in temperature is a significant sign of inflammation.[16] It's pretty hard for your fingers to pick up a one-degree temperature difference in a small area of the horse when the horse is sweating on a hot day. Looking for heat in the tissue, though interesting when it can be demonstrated, is only occasionally useful in making a diagnosis of lameness.

TESTING THE HOOF

As you will see, most lameness comes from the hoof. A device to test the hoof for sensitivity is therefore useful in lameness diagnosis. The "hoof testers" squeeze the foot. If the foot is sensitive, the horse will jump or pull the leg away from the device when it is applied. Interpretation of the results of hoof testing is something of an art. Some horses jump at anything. Conversely, an examiner can make just about any horse jump if he or she is strong enough. It sometimes helps to trot the horse before and after hoof tester application; if the horse is more lame after hoof testers are applied, you have an idea of where the source of the pain is. But again, since some horses will jump at anything, the application of hoof testers to a foot is another potential source for a lot of diagnostic error.

LOCAL ANESTHETIC BLOCKS

Local anesthetics are very commonly used to diagnose lameness. A horse limps because something hurts (obviously). If you make the area that hurts go numb, the horse stops limping. Thus, by injecting anesthetics into joints or above nerves in the horse's leg your veterinarian can get an idea of the location of the source of the pain.

This is not, of course, black and white (just like the rest of medicine). When anesthetics are injected over nerves, the area below the nerve goes numb. Just exactly what area has been anesthetized is not possible to determine accurately, although you can get a good idea of what's numb by poking around until the horse moves his leg away from the poke. It's very important to check the horse continually to make sure that what you think is numb is actually numb. The nerve supply to the leg of the horse has small individual variations for each horse. It's important to check that you haven't made more tissue numb than you thought. The anesthetic, though local, can spread after it's injected. If you don't recognize either of these circumstances, a mistake may be made in diagnosis. That being said, the use of anesthetics is very common in lameness examinations.[17,18]

You cannot determine the cause of a horse's lameness based solely on a response to anesthetic injection. Local anesthetic blocks only tell you the area that is sore. Suppose that a horse travels sound after his heels are blocked. You can't say that the horse has navicular disease or any other particular cause of heel lameness, for that matter; you can only say that the horse has sore heels. The quest for an accurate diagnosis of the cause of a horse's lameness requires further testing.

X RAYS

Radiographs, or X rays, are easy to take but harder to interpret. Interpretation takes training and experience. Your farrier and trainer should not be reading your horse's X rays, because although they are undoubtedly good people in their own right, they have absolutely no training in interpreting them. X rays are not "easy" to read.

X rays are a relatively imprecise and limited technique. They show only bone. They are not very useful for evaluating ligaments or tendons or nerves or other soft (nonbone) tissue. They also are not even a terribly accurate reflection of the state of the joints between the bone, as arthroscopic surgeons (who get to look directly into a joint) have shown. Radiographs can also vary between horses. Two completely different-looking X rays may be normal for each individual horse. In addition, "changes" from normal can be subtle. For these and other reasons, it is possible to get different opinions from two experts reading the same set of X rays.

The important thing about X rays is that they *can* be useful in helping to determine the root of a horse's lameness problem if the problem comes from the bone. If the problem doesn't relate to the bone, however, it's time to look at the leg with something else.

ULTRASOUND

Ultrasound has proven to be an effective way of looking inside horses, and it gives a look at some of the soft tissue. An ultrasound machine sends a sound wave into the tissue and analyzes the reflected sound that comes back. It's like using sonar to look for submarines in the ocean. Tissue reflects ultrasound back in different amounts, depending on its density, and this reflection is interpreted by a computer to give an image on the screen. Ultrasound is a marvelous way to look at the soft tissue of the horse's leg, but it doesn't penetrate bone.[19]

Of course, the use of ultrasound is by no means limited to the leg. By using different probes and different frequencies, a variety of internal structures can be visualized, such as the heart, kidneys and reproductive system.[20]

Unfortunately, like X rays, ultrasound is somewhat imprecise. The image obtained is related to the frequency of the beam required to get the image. The more tissue that has to be penetrated, the less clear the image that you look at is. Fortunately, in the legs, veterinarians are able to use an ultrasound beam that results in a fairly clear image since there isn't that much tissue to penetrate. This has enabled them to determine the extent of many (though not all) of a horse's soft tissue injuries with good accuracy.

In the diagnosis of tendon injuries, it is absolutely not possible to determine how badly your horse is injured without the use of ultrasound. Studies have shown that examining tendons while armed with nothing but experience and one's hands results in a missed diagnosis with alarming frequency. Therefore, anytime your horse has a lameness problem that results from an injury to one of the major tendons or ligaments of the lower leg, it's a good idea to have an ultrasound examination done. You'll feel better knowing how bad things are and how long healing of the injured tissue is going to take.

SCINTIGRAPHY

Scintigraphy has become an important diagnostic tool for some lame horses. This technique involves the injection of a radioactive substance into the horse's bloodstream. This substance then exits in areas of increased blood vessel permeability (where the blood vessels leak), such as in areas of inflammation. It can be a useful tool in helping to determine areas of inflammation or injury that are not readily identified by other techniques. It can be especially helpful in sorting out problems that occur in areas that are hard to examine, such as the pelvis or the horse's hoof.

Scintigraphy has unfortunately been touted by some as a quick and accurate way to pinpoint the source of a horse's lameness without having to actually work at the diagnostic process. That is, some people will tell you that with scintigraphy, a single shot of radioactive isotope will be able to diagnose all of the horse's ills. This just isn't the case. Scintigraphic examination is a fairly sensitive method of examination, but it is not terribly specific as to which tissue is involved. It should never be used as stated above, as a sort of instant whole-body lameness evaluator.

Scintigraphy does not give a direct image of tissue; it only shows inflammation. Scintigraphy should be used as an aid in diagnosis, in conjunction with other methods of lameness diagnosis. Scintigraphy, too, is a technique that is loaded with variations in interpretation. Though useful in many circumstances, this may also fail to tell you the cause of your horse's lameness.[21]

There are other tests and techniques employable in the diagnosis of lameness that may be applicable to particular situations. Some of these other tests are discussed in the chapter on legs. But even with all the things that veterinarians can do to try to identify the cause of lameness in a horse, sometimes the true underlying cause cannot be identified. You may be able to discover the area from which pain in the leg originates but you may *not* be able to determine the precise source of the pain. For example, it is not at all uncommon to have a horse with no soreness to palpation or hoof testers go sound when his heels are anesthetized. He may have normal X rays. A scintigraphic scan may not be helpful. When confronted with this unfortunate situation, you will have two choices.

One, you can realize that, unfortunately, some things cannot be diagnosed and some questions don't have answers. You will know that your horse probably doesn't have a broken bone. You may have to wait for some undetermined period of time until he begins to travel sound again. This requires patience.

Or, two, you can panic.

Panic occurs when your understandable desire to find out what's wrong with your horse gets the best of you and leads you to ask the advice of all sorts of trained, untrained and quasi-trained people. Thus, you will enter the worlds of chiropractors, helpful friends, psychics, kinesiologists and a whole host of others who will be only too happy to give you an opinion if you are willing to pay them for it. If you want something badly enough, you will be able to find someone to sell it to you. "Pseudodiagnosis" in horses is very easy, particularly since the horses can't contradict the diagnoser.

If you can't be patient or if you want a second opinion, get an expert one. If you are going to try something beyond traditional veterinary medicine, ask for some credentials. The least you can do for your good friend is be careful on his behalf.

2

Therapeutics

One of the natural instincts of humans is, evidently, to try to fix things that go wrong. Four hundred years ago, whenever someone was sick, the medical experts at the time were sure to have some sort of a cure. Just because humans didn't know how to cure themselves when they were sick didn't stop them from trying. The medical literature of the time talks about things like "bleeding" to cure diseases, in addition to a variety of other barbaric treatments.

Unfortunately, at least in the case of antiquated medical treatments, humans also have a good memory. This good memory for the things that used to be done, combined with a certain amount of nostalgia for the past, serves to ensure that older and all too frequently ineffective treatments will manage to sustain themselves. This problem is particularly troubling in equine therapeutics.

Therapeutics often seems to be based on a principle of opposites. That is, the therapy attempts to do the opposite of what is happening to the body. If something is hot, try to make it cold. If something swells, try to wrap it up. If something is "cold" (old and chronic), try to warm it up. If something is sticking out, try to stick it back in. Such general things are the goals of many treatments.

In many cases, treating by doing the opposite of what the body is doing is not a bad idea. But the treatment of any condition should be based on sound medical reasoning and not because it was what your dad used to do forty years ago.

Fortunately, therapeutic efforts are aided by one consistent principle: The body wants to heal. If tissue is injured in some way, the body will undertake considerable effort to try to repair the injury. The saying "Time heals all wounds" is particularly apt. Given enough time, the body will usually heal itself. Sometimes this healing is in spite of therapy (but the therapy generally gets the credit anyway).

Many things that are treated in horses are inflamed. Inflammation is a fascinating process that occurs in tissue when it is injured. It is not necessarily a bad thing; it is the inevitable consequence of injury. With inflammation comes the first stages of healing. Only when inflammation is uncontrolled (or uncontrollable) do problems arise.

(Infection is the result of the invasion and multiplication of foreign organisms, like bacteria or viruses, in the body. All infections result in inflammation of some sort, but not all inflamed tissue is infected.)

Inflammation, as it occurs in injured tissue, is a localized process that the body uses to protect itself. It is caused by injury to or destruction of body tissue. The process of inflammation serves to dilute, destroy or isolate both the injured tissue and the agent that caused the injury, allowing them to be removed or repaired.[1] Inflammation is usually a good thing.

When inflammation first occurs (acute inflammation) there are four classic signs that are seen in the horse: heat, pain, swelling and loss of function. On a microscopic level in the tissue, the events that occur with inflammation are very complicated and include a local dilation of the blood vessels and an increased ability of protein and cells to get out of the blood vessels (known as an increase in permeability of the vessels). The end result of all this activity is increased blood flow, increased protein and fluid and an increase in blood cells in the inflamed area.[2]

Even though the most commonly inflamed (and treated) areas in the horse are the legs, the general principles of the treatment of inflammation apply to all the body's tissues. The idea of providing therapy can be addressed rationally only if you understand what's going on inside.

HEAT

Heat in tissue is not a problem in and of itself. Heat is merely a sign of inflammation. It's not like the tissue is going to melt from being overheated. Heat in the tissue occurs because there is an increased volume of blood in the area of injury resulting from local vessel dilation. An area hot to the touch will generally be painful and uncomfortable. Applying cold to a hot area is a time-honored and medically useful way to relieve heat and associated pain from an inflamed area.

Although cooling a hot area may make an area more comfortable, cold on an acutely inflamed spot has other, even more beneficial, effects. Cold causes blood vessels to constrict. Blood vessels are not rigid tubes. They are made up of a bunch of cells tightly packed together in a tubular arrangement. When blood vessels are inflamed, spots where the cells are touching can begin to leak, allowing passage of fluid and cells into the tissue. If blood vessels in an inflamed area constrict due to cold, the gaps tend to close up. As a result, they cannot leak as much. This helps control swelling in an area, which has very positive effects.

Cold can be applied to a horse's leg via ice, a hose or a chemical ice pack and can be left on the leg for at least thirty minutes with no bad effects. By definition, acute inflammation doesn't last very long, and the application of cold doesn't need to be done for more than a couple of days at the most. Icing an injured leg every day for two weeks, while it demonstrates a remarkable concern for your horse, is also a waste of time. But putting cold on an acute hot spot is one time-honored method of treatment that really works.[3]

SWELLING

Leaky blood vessels let extra fluid, protein and cells into tissue. Since these things aren't in tissue in great amounts, the body makes room for them by swelling.

Swelling distorts the affected tissue. This has two bad effects. First, it causes pain. Swollen tissue gets all stretched out, and that hurts. Second, and perhaps more importantly, distortion of the tissue can increase the damage caused by the original injury. When tissue is torn by an injury, the swelling that occurs afterward has the potential to disrupt the integrity of the injured tissue even more, as the tissue stretches and spreads with the swelling. Thus, the control of swelling is very important, not only in the control of pain but also to prevent additional tissue injury.

In addition to cold, it also helps to apply pressure to a hot and swollen area. Pressure against a swollen area can help prevent it from swelling more. Obviously, if the pressure that is applied against the leg is greater than the pressure that is driving the fluid out of the blood vessels, the fluid won't be able to leave the vessels.[4] It is certainly possible to apply too much pressure to a swollen limb. Too much pressure is worse than not enough.

When horse owners see a swollen area on a horse, they tend to bandage it (if possible). It's kind of a knee-jerk reaction. But it's not a bad one. Bandaging is primarily done on the lower legs. After all, you can't very well bandage a horse's withers. Since the lower part of the horse's leg is roughly cylindrical, bandaging it isn't very difficult to do. As long as you don't try to pull the bandages too tight, you most likely will do it right, even if you do it sloppily. A variety of disposable and nondisposable products are just great for wrapping a leg, and they all work pretty well, assuming that the horse doesn't try to eat them.

"But wait!" your trainer screams. "You can't bandage the leg in *that* direction."

For some reason, horse people are terribly concerned about the "direction" in which the wrap should be applied. Should the wrap be applied clockwise or counterclockwise? Should the tendons be pulled to the inside or the outside of the leg? Should the bandage start at the top and go down or from the bottom and go up? What color should the bandage be? Why does everyone have a different answer to these questions?

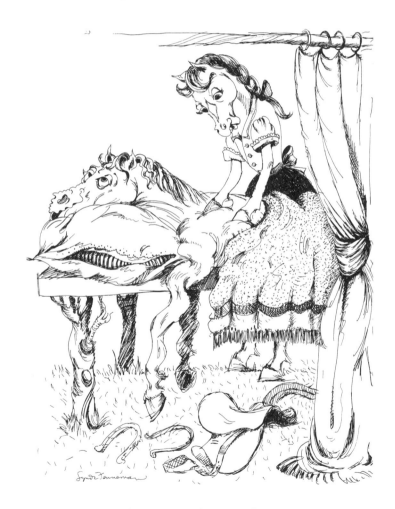

Therapeutic treatment can be important for a speedy recovery.

The direction of the wrap doesn't matter at all. There is absolutely no evidence or reason to believe that the direction of the wrap is important. If you ask enough people which particular direction is important and why, you will find that you won't get the same answer twice in a row.

Nor do you have to bandage the other leg if you bandage one. A horse does just fine with only one leg wrapped.

You can apply a bandage *poorly* if you are careless. A bandage that is applied too tightly, or slips down the leg, can constrict the horse's leg. This can result in an awful-looking swelling commonly called a bandage bow. (Fortunately, in the author's experience, these look a lot worse than they actually are, since it is rare that the underlying tendons get damaged.) As long as a bandage is applied with a moderate amount of tension; as long as you are not seeing how tightly you can wrap a leg; as long as you change the wrap occasionally to prevent pressure spots from popping up—you are unlikely to do anything bad to your horse's leg. And the direction certainly doesn't matter.

Don't be mad at your friends when they tell you to wrap a leg in the "only" correct method. They're trying to be helpful. Just don't listen to them.

PAIN

Because acutely inflamed tissue is injured, swollen and hot, it is also quite painful. If you manipulate a swollen and inflamed joint or tendon of the horse's leg, he will let you know that it hurts. If you can find this area of heat, pain and swelling, you are on your way to attaining a diagnosis (and understanding the career of a veterinarian).

The control of pain can be very important in the treatment of inflammation, if only for humane reasons. After all, there is no reason why your horse should stand around and hurt. Indeed, if pain is such a problem that the horse is not using his leg, or, as in a case of abdominal pain (colic), is thrashing around, the pain itself has the potential to cause serious complications. In the case of a leg injury, for example, it is possible for a horse to break down in an otherwise unaffected leg if all of his weight is borne on the "good" leg for too long. In the case of the colicking horse, he can hurt himself by rolling around while trying to get comfortable (he will not twist his intestines, as you will read later). Controlling heat and swelling will also help control pain. All of these things occur together.

Anti-inflammatory and pain-relieving agents will help counteract the pain of inflammation. In the treatment and control of acute pain and inflammation, these drugs are of great benefit when used properly and have few bad effects.

Just because your horse limps a little bit at the trot doesn't mean that you have to give him a pain reliever. Pain control should not be undertaken indiscriminately. The presence of minor pain can be a very useful indicator of recovery from an injury. (This is not cruel.) After acute inflammation and pain are controlled, it is frequently advisable to discontinue pain-relieving drugs. While your horse is on these drugs, an otherwise painful stimulus may be covered up. As a result, you may not be able to tell if your horse is improving. If you want to see if your horse is really getting better, make sure that he is drug free when you're looking at him.

LOSS OF FUNCTION

Just as loss of function is a sign of acute inflammation, return to function is a sign that the inflammation is subsiding. Loss of function can occur as a result of pain (which makes the horse not want to use the leg), or as a result of swelling or the degree of tissue injury (which makes the horse unable to use the leg). By applying the above-mentioned techniques to help control acute inflammation, you do the best you can to help ensure that a horse will regain full function as soon as possible.

CHRONIC INFLAMMATION

Chronic inflammation is a more difficult and troubling problem than acute inflammation. Chronic inflammation is inflammation that progresses slowly. It may result from the continuation of an acute condition or a prolonged low-grade condition. Chronic inflammation is highlighted primarily by the formation of new tissue. It usually causes permanent tissue damage.[1]

As new tissue forms in chronic inflammation, the function of the old tissue can be disrupted. For example, in a joint, as inflammation progresses (arthritis) new bone is formed. This new bone in the joint is a source of chronic pain and dysfunction, and you can't make it go away.[5] In tendons, as inflammation progresses, scar tissue forms. This new tissue enlarges the tendon and may attach itself to other tissues. This can disrupt the normal ability of the tendons to glide along next to each other.[6] In the abdomen, chronic inflammation can cause the intestines to stick to each other. The new tissue that is produced can cause scarring and adhesions that impede the normal propulsive movements of the bowel.[7]

Chronic inflammation is difficult if not impossible to cure. The new tissue that is formed can generally not be removed so that the affected tissue can be returned to normal. Consequently, therapeutic efforts are frequently aimed at the control of chronic inflammation and at trying to make the affected horse as comfortable as possible while having to live with it.

A chronically inflamed area does not have much heat in the tissue and is commonly said to be cold. Based on the "principle of opposites," how do you think that chronic inflammation is most commonly treated (in the leg, anyway)? By trying to make the area hot, of course!

This trying to make cold tissue warm must come from the way human beings deal with their own bodies. In people with a sore, arthritic joint or a stiff back muscle, the application of some form of heat, via direct application of a hot pad, a counterirritant rub or even a good hot soak can help loosen up a chronically inflamed area. Is it the same in horses?

They'll never tell.

You'll never stop trying.

Some of the things that are done to warm up cold areas in horses makes some good medical sense. For instance, it is well known that horses will often warm up out of minor stiffness with exercise. As a chronically inflamed joint or muscle functions, the function usually does improve. Indeed, it is thought that limited exercise is of benefit in the treatment and control of chronic inflammation of joints. This helps prevent stiffness and dysfunction (among other positive benefits) and probably should be encouraged.[8,9] The application of counterirritants and rubs to your horse may be useful in helping to warm up a stiff area, too. In people, locally applied counterirritants (there are a bunch of them on the shelf at your drugstore) will cause surface blood vessels to dilate and make the tissue feel warmer and "looser" for a while. They *may* do the same thing for horses.

Another effective way to keep the temperature of an area elevated is by bandaging it. Bandaging insulates the tissue and helps retain heat. Consequently, many horses with chronic lower leg stiffness are bandaged all the time.

Therapeutic efforts in the chronically inflamed leg also try to relieve the pain that occurs as a result of the abnormal tissue. The use of anti-inflammatory and pain-relieving drugs again becomes important in treating horses so afflicted. Since chronic conditions usually cannot be cured, horses with chronic inflammation often have to be on therapeutic doses of these drugs for a long time. (In the same manner, human patients with chronic arthritis usually are on the same type of drugs indefinitely.) Long-term use of these drugs is generally safe for horses.

"Increasing the Circulation"

There is a huge amount of therapeutic effort directed at "improving" or "increasing" the circulation to a healing area, so that it can heal better. What does this mean? Increasing the circulation would have to mean that the volume of blood to an area goes up. This could only be done in a limited number of ways, either by dilation of the local blood vessels (which would allow more blood to get to the area) or by increasing the number of blood vessels in an area (same effect) or by increasing the speed of delivery of the blood (by increasing the rate at which the heart pumps). Anyway, according to those who promote this idea, if the circulation can be increased, healing will increase, too.

Certainly, if there is no circulation to an area, bad things happen. An area without circulation won't heal. In fact, it will probably fall off the body. Just because not enough circulation is bad, however, doesn't mean that more circulation is good, or even possible. In fact, *no one has ever demonstrated that any method of therapy can "increase" circulation to any area of the horse.* Furthermore, *no one has ever shown that if circulation of blood to an area could be increased, it would increase healing anyway.* This is really hard to believe. But it's true. Although an "increase in circulation" is the therapeutic goal of a terrific number of medical and quasi-medical therapies, so far no one has ever shown that it can be done, much less that it would do any good if it could be done! Paradoxically, many chronically inflamed areas *have* an increase in the number of blood vessels to them. The "increased circulation" in these areas can be part of the problem. Keep these facts in mind the next time someone talks to you about "improving" or "increasing" circulation. In spite of all of these facts, however, there are all sorts of devices and therapies for horses that purport to increase circulation. There are old and barbaric forms of therapies like firing and blistering. There are new and humane devices like lasers, electromagnetic devices, regular magnetic devices and therapeutic ultrasound.

The problem with the new devices, at least from a medical standpoint, is that so far none of them has shown the ability to do anything to affect healing in a consistent or repeatable fashion. Some therapies have shown some beneficial effects on some tissues in some species (sometimes). Unfortunately, the majority of them have had limited study in the horse. The results of a test on one species may not be applicable to another, either. For example, the data from a study on ultrasound and tendon healing in the toe of a chicken may not necessarily be applicable to the horse.[10] Those studies that have been done on horses often show inconsistent results, or no effect whatsoever.[11,12,13,14]

Modern machines and old forms of therapy persist primarily because of anecdotal reports. You know, your friend's grandfather did it that way. Or, "lots of horses have been helped" by a particular form of therapy. Or, "more trainers use . . . " to keep their horses running stronger. Surprisingly little research has been done to document all of the good effects that the more modern and mysterious therapeutic devices supposedly provide.

While people's intentions are most likely good when they try to treat horses, just because a horse seems to improve after a particular therapy has started doesn't mean that the therapy caused the improvement. Just because *b* follows *a* doesn't mean that *b* was caused by *a*. Don't waste your time or money on futile attempts at therapy that are unproven, unlikely to work and expensive. Your laudable wishes to help heal your horse shouldn't be blinded by the fact that someone out there may want to take advantage of you and sell you something.

Before trying out any new therapeutic device, look for good, solid data to support it. Just ask for the facts and skip the fluff. If there were any miracles to be had, you can be sure that the veterinary community would be at the forefront of trying to promote them; everybody wants hurt horses to get better. Go into these newer forms of treatment with your eyes open. While everyone would love to have something that made healing faster, better and stronger, if it existed everyone would be using it, not only in horses but in people, too.

And stop trying to "increase" your horse's circulation.

Only one thing "increases" circulation to an area by dilating local blood vessels. That thing is inflammation. Why would you want this? Think about it. Inflammation is a response to injury by the body. To make the body better, you damage it, right? Right?

Did you really believe your mother when she said that the medicine must do some good because it tasted so bad?

But believe it or not, you will hear some people promoting acute inflammation as a cure for chronic inflammation. That is, they advise making a chronically inflamed area acutely inflamed in the hope that healing will occur after the acute inflammation subsides.[15] This method is mentioned in a book published in 1832 that is in the author's collection.[16] It's hard to believe that this sort of therapeutic objective is still brought up, particularly since we have come as far as we have in other areas (like flush toilets and home mail service). But it is one of the justifications for outmoded and archaic treatments like firing and blistering. It doesn't work.

FIRING AND BLISTERING

Firing and blistering are inhumane forms of "therapy" that have been around for literally hundreds of years. The underlying basis for this type of treatment is, you guessed it, to get more circulation to the affected area.

Blistering is the application of an extremely irritating substance to the skin. This irritation will be so extreme, say the proponents, that the tissue will become acutely inflamed. Therefore, say the blisterers, more blood will come into the area and increase the healing of the underlying tissue. Or, say some other proponents, it will cause a layer of scar tissue to be laid down over the injured tissue that will strengthen and support it.

Firing is supposed to work the same way as blistering. The only difference is that it is a more severe treatment. When a horse is fired, his legs are anesthetized first because the next step is to take a red-hot firing iron and burn holes in his skin. This is done in one of a variety of innovative and decorative patterns. When the procedure is finished, your horse will have bleeding holes in his legs and his legs *will* become very inflamed.

These procedures have two things in common. First of all, they cause the horse intense pain. Second, they don't do anything to promote circulation, healing or anything else. It has been well demonstrated that firing serves only to inflame and scar the skin and does nothing for the underlying tissues that are supposed to be the targets of this type of therapy (and in fact hurts them). The "increased" circulation occurs only in the skin that has been acutely and severely inflamed by the treatment.[17] Scar tissue is *always* weaker than normal tissue and doesn't function to strengthen anything. These "therapies" are barbaric and archaic and—in the author's opinion, as well as that of the American Humane Society—have no place in the treatment of horse injuries.

The only thing that these therapies do is to enforce rest in an injured horse. If you cannot accept the fact that your injured horse will need time to heal and you have to hurt him further to give him that time, shame on you.

CHIROPRACTIC

Chiropractic is a system of therapeutics in human medicine that is based on the claim that disease is caused by abnormal function of the nerve system.[1] It attempts to restore normal nerve system function by manipulation and treatment of body tissues, especially those of the spine. Studies of chiropractic in humans indicate some benefit from manipulation, although that benefit may be only from massage.

There are big problems in the veterinary community with the idea of chiropractic as applied to horses. Due to the size and mass of the vertebrae, muscles and associated ligaments in and around the spinal column of the horse (you are talking about fist-sized vertebrae through muscle and ligament that's often a foot thick or more), it seems unlikely that effective manipulation or movement is even possible. Certainly, to this point no one has shown it is. Chiropractors cannot directly demonstrate where a problem is (by taking X rays, for example), nor can they show you that they have corrected the "problem."

There is a training program in veterinary chiropractic that certifies veterinarians who have been trained in chiropractic manipulation. If you choose this sort of therapy, you should at least make sure that the person who is doing it is certified by the IVCA.[19] Call them. The field is full of people who represent themselves as chiropractors who have no training in chiropractic, animal anatomy, disease diagnosis or anything else. Furthermore, a human chiropractor doesn't necessarily know what he or she is doing on an animal. Untrained personnel can often create problems or even make things worse.

According to the head of the International Veterinary Chiropractic Association (IVCA), the sound or loud "pop" that can sometimes be heard with manipulation of the horse has nothing to do with "adjusting" the spine and does not necessarily indicate success. Don't be fooled by a sound into thinking that something is happening. Chiropractic is a series of specific movements; you cannot adjust a whole horse by backing him in the corner or pulling on his tail. You should also be very suspicious of anyone who uses mallets or two-by-four blocks of wood to assist in adjustments; these are not needed.[18] Chiropractic does not replace diagnosis. It is a treatment method that is in infancy.

If someone starts to hammer on your horse's back or jerk hard on his tail in an effort to "straighten" his vertebrae, be careful. Don't let your friend get hurt. Chiropractic is an area that cries out for research to be done to see what, if any, effect can be attained by manipulation of the horse. Since there are no studies of this form of treatment, it is very difficult to determine what benefit can be had from equine chiropractic.

ACUPUNCTURE

Acupuncture is a completely different way to look at the body. It is, of course, commonly practiced in Asia.

The differences in thought between Western and Eastern medicine can be quite dramatic. For instance, in Western medicine it is thought that when the heart pumps, the blood moves. In Eastern medicine it is felt that the energy flow caused by the blood moving causes the heart to beat. Acupuncture purports to affect the flow of energy through the body by the use of needles placed at specific points.[1] Animal studies have shown that acupuncture can be an effective way of relieving pain and even inducing local anesthesia. Other claims, such as the healing of medical conditions in animals, cannot be supported. But the fact remains that if your horse is suffering from acute or chronic pain or inflammation, acupuncture may be an effective way to provide some relief for him. It is one of the things that you can consider in treating a difficult condition or one that is not responsive to traditional therapies.[20] There are training programs in veterinary acupuncture. If you elect to use this form of therapy, you should employ someone who has completed this training.

OTHER THERAPIES

Some of the things that are done to horses in an effort to help them are fascinating. No one has any idea if they work or not. Frequently they are done because they "should" work. Most of these things can't possibly do any harm to your horse, but when you stop and think about them you wonder.

Take soaking a horse's foot. In the case of a recently opened abscess, soaking a foot may do some good, if only because it keeps the area clean while it is trying to heal. But does soaking help soothe a bruised foot? Certainly, if *your* feet are sore, a good hot soak makes them feel better. But is it the same with your horse? Who knows? Chances are, you will go on soaking anyway. At the very least, it will make you feel like you are doing something good for your horse, no matter how much he doesn't like it.

What about poultices and cataplasms? They are applied to a horse's legs in an effort to soothe or to "draw out" abscesses or inflammation or swellings. Poultices generate heat in tissue. In humans, this can cause some soothing and muscle relaxation. But does it do anything for horses when it's put on their feet or legs? No one knows.

The idea of drawing out an abscess is certainly a bit odd and unlikely. It's unclear how putting something on the skin or the hoof could influence the direction in which an abscess will expand. Poultices allegedly draw fluid to the surface because their high concentration of material (osmotic tension) is supposed to suck fluid to it, like throwing salt on top of ice.[21]

You would hope that anything that you put on the skin to draw out bad stuff would stay on top of the skin on the epidermis. If it didn't stay on the top of the skin, it would be absorbed into the bloodstream. Most poultices are made of clay, which, if absorbed into the bloodstream, would kill the horse! But since the skin is not a barrier that is freely and easily penetrated, putting something on it doesn't mean that anything underneath it will be affected. Abscesses, as they grow, will always expand toward the area of least resistance. It's unlikely that softening the skin or hoof or trying to make it more moist will have any significant effect on hastening the opening of the abscess, since the skin and surface areas of the hoof are generally the softest areas around. Don't get too excited about trying to draw toxins or abscesses.

Sweat wraps are frequently applied to horse legs to reduce swelling. An occlusive dressing, like petrolatum, glycerin or a water-based antibiotic, is applied to the skin in a thick layer. The leg is then wrapped in plastic and bandaged. When the bandage is removed, the swelling will frequently be reduced or be gone altogether.

This effect is well known, but why it actually occurs is anyone's guess. Most likely some local dehydrating effect on the skin from this type of wrap reduces some swelling, at least temporarily. The effect these wraps produce may be simply due to the counterpressure applied by the bandaging.[22] Why some of these things work is part of the charm and mystery of equine therapeutics.

TIME AS THERAPY

The most important form of therapy that you can give your horse is time. If a horse is sick or injured and the problem can be repaired, it will take time to heal. The time to heal may seem interminable. You will go nuts because you can't go riding. You will want the horse to heal faster than he can, but you have to be patient.

"I know the bone is sticking out, Doc, but I have a horse show in two weeks."

Please.

Horses cannot heal any faster than people, or any other animal for that matter. If a football player hurts a ligament in his knee, with surgery, time for healing and time for rehabilitation, he may be able to return to full function in many months, depending on the severity of the injury. If he starts back too soon he can hurt himself all over again and flush all of the time and therapy down the drain.

It's the same with a horse: healing of tissue takes time. The best thing that you can give your horse, in addition to your good care, is the time that it takes for something to heal. If you can provide time for healing to occur, many things will take care of themselves, in spite of what everyone else says you "have" to do.

One final point about therapy in horses. Sometimes, therapy is more for the benefit of the horse owner than the horse. Your veterinarian may be called to see a problem in your horse that you are sure requires some form of therapy, say, a small bump on the side of his neck. After examining the horse, the veterinarian may well determine that the bump is inconsequential, does not threaten the horse's health or well-being and can be left alone.

You want it treated because you hate it.

Your friends hate it, too.

You all agree that something *has* to be done.

Who's getting treated here, anyway?

The point is, many things in horses may not need therapy at all. At times, therapy for a horse may be directed at soothing the owner, since the problem doesn't bother the horse. The horse doesn't care if he has a bump on his neck. *His* friends won't notice or laugh at him. But if you feel better rubbing or icing or applying some sort of goo on top of your horse's bump, your horse most likely won't mind too much. Who knows, *you* may feel much better taking care of the horse, so maybe it's not such bad therapy after all.

Of course, there are many other therapies for specific conditions in the horse. Antibiotics kill infections and intravenous fluids help relieve dehydration, for example. The search for new forms of therapy is continuous. Though occasionally breakthroughs do occur, unfortunately they are not very common. Most forms of therapies should make some sort of sense and should be relatively easy for you to understand, at least in principle. There's nothing wrong with wanting to "do something" for your horse, even if he doesn't really have much of a problem. But always remember, the most important principle of any therapy is to "do no harm." When things get weird, watch out.

3

Drugs

Since the dawn of time we have tried to make health problems better with medicines. Medicine men (and women—many of the early healers were women) ground up herbs and plants to make powders and applied the powders and plants directly to problem areas. As medicine men evolved they became known as pharmacologists. These people studied and analyzed these powders and their effects and purified them and saw that they were good. Then they hired professionals to sell, advertise and market them, and soon they were big business.

Fortunately, the drugs and medications that evolved tend to be good. One of the most baffling myths is that therapeutic drugs are somehow bad or unnatural. Without question, ingesting a foreign substance is going to result in some sort of effect on your horse's body. That's the point; you are looking for some sort of effect from the drug. In many cases, this effect is much more desirable than the natural alternative, say, death from a bacterial infection that could otherwise have been treated. Most drugs, when given at the manufacturer's recommended doses, are safe and frequently effective.

If you are dead set against giving your horse any drugs or foreign substances, at least be consistent. Don't deworm him, don't give him medications if he gets sick, don't give him pain relievers if he gets sore, don't nail shoes on his feet, let his teeth grow long and sharp and don't give him processed "unnatural" feeds. Good luck.

If, however, you are interested in what is done to horses with various drugs and medications, read on.

32

ADMINISTERING THE DRUG

Before discussing types of drugs, you should know how drugs are given to horses. Usually drugs are given in one of three ways: orally, intramuscularly or intravenously. How a drug is administered is absolutely critical. Phenylbutazone, for instance, in its injectable form, must be given intravenously. The stuff is very irritating to tissue if given in the muscle and can cause nasty muscle abscesses. Penicillin, as another example, is very poorly absorbed if given orally and thus must be given by one of the other means.[1] Remember, for a drug to work and not hurt your horse, it's critical that it be given by the proper route.

Ultimately, for any drug to work, it has to be absorbed into the horse's bloodstream. The drug will then circulate through the bloodstream and arrive at its intended destination where, ideally, it will produce the desired effect. (Incidentally, if the bloodstream doesn't get to an area, like the center of an abscess or the abdominal cavity, it can be very difficult to get drugs to the site and cause any effect.) Meanwhile, since the drug is a foreign substance, the body is working furiously trying to remove it. Consequently, when talking about the effects of drugs on the horse's system, it is important to know how long the drug is going to stay there. In order to quantify this amount of time, pharmacologists talk about how long it takes for one half of the drug to be removed from the horse. This is known as the half-life of the drug.

One of the most common myths involved in the administration of a drug is that if you double the dose, you will double the effect.

"Boy, he's really lame. Let's give him four pills instead of two."

If you double the dose of a drug, you only increase the amount given by one half-life. Or, to put it another way, you increase the length of time that a dose will stay in the system by one half-life. For example, let's say the half-life of a drug is four hours, about what it is for phenylbutazone, the most commonly given pain reliever in horses. A frequently prescribed dose of this drug for a thousand-pound horse is two grams every twelve hours. If you double the dose to four grams, after one half-life there will be two grams left, since half of the original four-gram dose will be gone. Therefore, by doubling the dose of the drug, you only increase the time that the drug stays in the system by four hours. Thus, after only four hours, you are right back to the recommended initial drug dose anyway.

While doubling the dose of a drug will not significantly increase the effectiveness, it very effectively increases the potential for side effects for some drugs, such as phenylbutazone.[2] You should always follow the recommended dosage of a drug, as given to you by your veterinarian and not your farrier, horse trainer or best friend.

The way that a drug is given to the horse affects how it works. The route of administration of a drug affects two things: (1) How rapidly the drug gets into the bloodstream and (2) what blood level of the drug is ultimately reached. These two things are generally directly related; that is, the more quickly a substance gets into the bloodstream, the higher the level that is reached.

The fastest way to get a substance into the bloodstream is, obviously, to shoot it right on in. Thus, the intravenous route of administration, when appropriate, provides the most rapid, most easily controlled and highest circulating blood level of a drug that can be attained. The highest level that can be attained, however, does not also ensure the "best" effect, only that it will get into the blood right away.

The intramuscular route of administration is sort of a middle ground. When a drug is given in the muscle, it is absorbed into the bloodstream more slowly than if the drug is given in the vein. By this route, the level of the drug never gets as high as that which is attained by intravenous administration, but it may get high enough to be effective. Also, because drugs are absorbed more slowly when given in the muscle, they tend to stay in the circulation longer than when given in the vein. Drug preparations can even be made so that they are hard for the body to absorb. When given in the muscle, these preparations release the drug slowly and consequently prolong its effect.

The oral route of administration of a drug is similar to the intramuscular route in that it tends to produce a lower, longer-lasting level of a drug than does the intravenous route. Certain drugs are only given orally, but others cannot be. This is because when a drug is given orally, it is not directly absorbed by the bloodstream. A drug can be dramatically affected by the stomach or intestines, or even not allowed to pass through these barriers at all.[3]

Medications applied directly on the surface of the horse, such as in the eye, generally have no measurable effect on the horse's system. However, if a medication is applied to an open wound, it can *potentially* be absorbed.

One thing that all routes of drug administration have in common in horses is that horses usually hate them. Most horses understandably tire rapidly of being jabbed with sharp needles. They can be quite particular about what you try to hide in their feed, too. And if you squirt something into their mouth, they are not at all shy about trying to spit it out. Drug administration to the horse can be quite a challenge and a big mess, too. One of the nice things about intramuscular or intravenous administration of drugs is that the horse will get the entire dose, however unpleasant the experience is for both of you. If you are giving oral medication, it is particularly important to make sure that the horse is getting the entire dose if you expect a good result from treatment.

Making sure that the horse is getting the entire dose of an oral medication is ever so much easier said than done, of course. If you are lucky, your horse will not be a discriminating eater and will happily gobble up whatever sort of pill or powder you mix with his feed. More likely, he will manage to nibble up every little trace of feed and leave a nice little pile of medication sitting forlornly in his feeder. Or he may just decide not to eat any feed at all.

There are dozens of ways to try to get your horse to take oral medication. You can mix the medication with honey, molasses, pancake syrup, soft drinks, grain, bran or beer until you are blue in the face and your horse may still decline to eat it. By the time you've tried everything, you may have to get another bottle of medication to replace what you've just wasted.

Fortunately, many medications come in a paste form, just like deworming products, and you can usually get them in the horse's mouth. Patience and good luck to you.

That being said, there is this bizarre phenomenon that sometimes occurs when drugs are prescribed. Many times, no matter what the route of administration, the drugs don't work at all. This is not a myth. This is because it has been estimated that 50 percent of all drugs that are prescribed are never given. What is even more amazing is that frequently the people who are not giving the drugs are also baffled that the horse isn't getting better. Sometimes the horse gets better anyway, despite lack of treatment, but that's beside the point. If you want your horse to get the full effects of his drugs, *give* them to him. If you have problems with administering them, tell your vet. There's nothing to be ashamed of because your horse doesn't want to take his medication.

ANTIBIOTICS AND ANTIBACTERIALS

Antibiotics come from naturally occurring substances, like molds or plants. Antibacterials are substances that are manufactured. Both substances attempt to kill bacteria. Most people call everything used to fight infection antibiotics; it's really a matter of semantics.

Antibiotics have revolutionized medicine since their introduction about fifty years ago. These drugs have a variety of clever ways to kill or control the growth of bacteria. Unfortunately, bacteria are relatively adept at finding new and clever ways to avoid being killed or controlled, so the development of new antibiotics is one of the many things that keeps drug companies in business.

If your horse gets an infection, he may be a candidate for treatment with antibiotics. Under most circumstances, antibiotics do not eliminate infections. Rather, they kill or control the growth of enough bacteria until such time as the horse's immune system is able to take charge and clean up the infectious mess. If a horse is really sick, antibiotic therapy may have to be more aggressive (using multiple antibiotics or ones that kill a wide range of bacteria) or more prolonged than if an infection is relatively minor.

That being said, it has been estimated that 70 percent of all infections will be taken care of by the body if nothing at all is done.[1] The problem, of course, is that there's no way to tell just by looking at the horse if he is one of the 70 percent or one of the other 30 percent that will eventually need help. Thus, most horses with infections will get treated with antibiotics, "just in case."

Not all infections are caused by bacteria, however. In fact, most respiratory infections are not caused by bacteria. They are caused by viruses, just like colds in people.

Viruses aren't killed by antibiotics. Almost nothing kills a virus, so the person who ends the search for drugs to control viruses effectively is going to be very rich and famous. Still, antibiotics are very commonly administered to any horse with an infection, even if the infection is caused by a virus.

The rationale for this is that the virus may somehow weaken the host system and allow the development of a secondary bacterial infection in the already diseased tissue. By giving antibiotics, the story goes, you can prevent the secondary infection until the body has time to mount an immune response and fight off the virus on its own.

Medically this sounds great, but the ground on which this argument is built is quite shaky. There is a lot of discussion in the medical community about how important this secondary infection phenomenon is in real life. There is little strong evidence that it is a frequent occurrence. Also, there is some evidence that the indiscriminate use of antibiotics creates strains of bacteria that resist being killed by almost anything. Thus, the fear is that by giving antibiotics to every sick animal some sort of "super" bacteria will be created that will be nothing but trouble.

Bacteria, like everything else, like to live. If you give antibiotics to a horse with a bacterial infection, ideally the vast majority of the bad bacteria will be killed. The survivors, however, can continue to grow in spite of the antibiotics, and they will grow and reproduce happily. To kill these bacteria, a second drug may be needed, and if some of these bacteria survive the second drug, you now have a growing bacteria that is resistant to two antibiotics. Furthermore, bacteria have ways of transferring their acquired resistance to other bacteria. The whole thing gets quite complex.

Also, you need bacteria in your horse's body, for things like digestion. The indiscriminate use of antibiotics also has the potential to affect adversely the population of "good" bacteria in your horse and allow for an overgrowth of

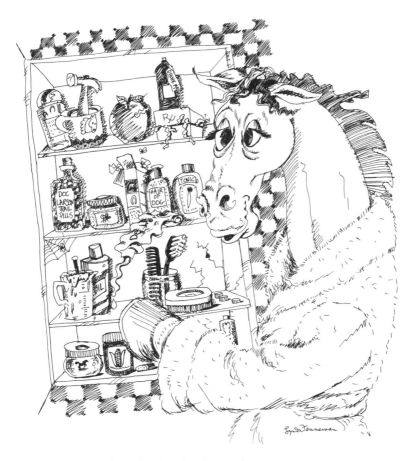

The right drug for the right situation is very important.

"bad" bacteria. As a practical matter, this is very uncommon in horses, but it is a big problem in human medicine.

So what does all this mean? Like most everything else in medicine, there is rarely a black and white answer. If your horse gets an infection, antibiotics are often a useful way to get rid of it. But you should be aware that the use of antibiotics is not necessarily benign and that every little jump in your horse's temperature or bit of nasal discharge does not require an antibiotic response from you. Don't just run to a feed store and start dumping penicillin into your sick horse. Check with your veterinarian first. The selection of a proper antibiotic is important. Diagnostic tests, such as attempting to isolate and grow bacteria to see which antibiotics are most effective, may be recommended. Some infections may not require antibiotics at all, and some things that you think are infections may not be, either. Lots of factors are involved in making what appears, on the surface, to be a relatively simple decision to give antibiotics to your horse.

Antibiotics are surprisingly free of side effects in horses, although side effects can occur. Sure, horses can develop allergies to antibiotics such as penicillin or develop kidney problems from the aminoglycoside group, just like people. There are no emergency warning bracelets for horses, so make sure you don't forget if your horse has or develops a problem with an antibiotic.

Other factors can affect the toxicity of antibiotics. If a horse is really sick, the time that it takes for these (or any) drugs to be removed from the system may be prolonged because of his depressed metabolism. It may be important to monitor him for bad side effects (especially those that affect the kidneys) when antibiotics are used. Antibiotic (in fact most drug) doses may also be different in baby horses. Immature animals have immature kidneys and livers. Antibiotics can affect them differently than adults. Your veterinarian will undoubtedly want to monitor such things as kidney function and drug levels if your horse is really sick, to make sure that the drugs themselves aren't hurting your horse.

Remember that antibiotics must be used judiciously and properly. They are wonderful drugs that will help your horse through a lot of problems.

ANTI-INFLAMMATORIES AND PAIN RELIEVERS

Among the most commonly prescribed drugs for horses are anti-inflammatories and pain relievers.

They are divided into two broad classes of drugs, steroidal and nonsteroidal types. (The term "steroid" refers to a chemical configuration.)

STEROIDS

"Steroid" is also used to apply to a type of drug known as an anabolic steroid. These are the drugs that get so much press about their abuse in weight lifters, track stars and football players. This is a different type of drug (although chemically similar) and will not be discussed here.

Steroidal anti-inflammatory drugs are very useful drugs. They come in long-lasting and short-lasting varieties. These drugs are very potent relievers of inflammation and have a variety of uses in equine medicine. They do not relieve pain, however, as do the nonsteroidal drugs. They can be used in the treatment of allergic reactions, shock and inflammation.

Steroids are very similar to substances that occur in the body of the horse (and in our own bodies). In most species, when steroids are taken in from an outside source, the body slows or shuts down production of its own natural substances. Then, when the drug is withdrawn, the body can find itself in a bit of trouble if there is no natural production going on. The body needs the drug in *some* form.

Therefore, in most species, when steroids are withdrawn, it is generally done so over a period of time. The dose of the drug is decreased gradually so the body can get the hint that the outside source is being withdrawn and resume production on its own.

People hate steroids, especially if they have taken them or have had a dog or cat that did. In dogs, cats and people, steroids make the patient want to eat, drink and urinate. Small animals and people tend to get fat and bloated on these drugs and the body becomes dependent on them.

For some reason, horses are different. They can be maintained on large doses of these drugs for long periods of time and then withdrawn immediately with no apparent ill effects. Nobody understands why this is so, but in this regard steroids are actually a much safer drug for horses than they are in other species.

Yet one bad side effect is *occasionally* seen when steroids are given to the horse: laminitis (founder), a serious condition that causes inflammation of the connection between the live hoof tissue and the hoof itself. To decrease the chances of this happening, it is generally felt that short-acting steroids should be used, when possible, instead of long-acting ones and that horses should also be kept on the drugs for as short a time as possible. Contrary to what you might hear, this does not occur very often, so don't be afraid to employ these drugs if they are needed. As you might imagine, steroids should *never* be used in the treatment of laminitis.[2]

Steroids are also commonly employed in the treatment of joint inflammation. The drugs are injected directly into an inflamed joint and are very effective in reducing all of the signs that are associated with inflammation. Used judiciously, these drugs are not harmful, do not hurt the joint cartilage and are not associated with future joint problems, assuming the injected joint did not have any serious underlying damage.[4,5]

The use of steroids in the joint has been implicated in causing problems in joints that are already damaged, however. When injected into a damaged joint, steroids may actually exacerbate an injury in the long term, even if they provide some immediate short-term relief. Over time, steroids in a damaged joint may promote further damage by suppressing the body's attempts at repairing the joint. They can thereby indirectly accelerate joint destruction. Thus, the use of these drugs in a joint, while often helpful at relieving inflammation, should also not be indiscriminate.[4]

Many health conditions warrant the use of steroids in the horse. Although anti-inflammatory steroids in the joint have come under fire for being responsible for any number of negative effects on horse limbs, much of the time the criticism isn't valid. Don't believe that these are bad drugs. Like all drugs, use them wisely and follow directions and your horse will be just fine.

NONSTEROIDAL ANTI-INFLAMMATORIES

The other class of anti-inflammatory drugs is the nonsteroidals, which are among the most widely used drugs in medicine. Drugstores stock them for human use, and drugs such as aspirin, ketoprofen, phenylbutazone, flunixin meglumine and meclofenamic acid are all nonsteroidals that are used in horses. Fortunately, the trade names of these drugs are usually easier to pronounce than the generic names.

Phenylbutazone ("bute") is the most frequently prescribed drug in this class. It is prescribed because it works and because it's pretty cheap. With the exception of aspirin, none of the other drugs even approaches cheap.

Nonsteroidal anti-inflammatory drugs have two effects on the horse. As the name suggests, they relieve inflammation (and all of the things that go with it, such as heat and swelling). As such, they are tremendously useful in treating acute and chronic injuries in a variety of tissues. Unlike steroids, this group of drugs also helps control pain and reduce fevers.

These drugs are commonly used long term in the treatment and control of chronic inflammation. In a horse with a chronic injury, it is not always possible to effect a cure and to return the horse to full, normal function. The use of anti-inflammatory pain-relieving drugs may allow this horse to continue to function more normally and free of pain.

"But wait," you cry. "You're just covering up the problem!"

Well, yes.

Frequently, the alternative to the use of pain-relieving, anti-inflammatory drugs in controlling chronic inflammation is to stop using the horse. If you have a horse with a chronic, incurable condition, you may be faced with a philosophical decision. You may have to choose between whether you want to continue to use the horse, knowing that his condition is only being "covered up" by the drug, or whether you want to stop using the horse. His condition may continue to get a bit worse while he is kept relatively pain free. Without the drugs, he may not be able to perform at all. You *can* begin to try to find another horse. Sometimes other considerations besides those that are strictly medical are very important, you see.

Nonsteroidal anti-inflammatory drugs control pain by interfering with the chemical pathways by which a pain-causing chemical, prostaglandin, is formed. There is a complex series of chemical reactions that result in the formation of these chemicals by the body. Each of the nonsteroidal pain-relieving drugs tries to prevent the formation of these chemicals in a different way. Some drugs may work better than others for certain conditions.[2,6]

Nonsteroidals get something of a bad reputation for a couple of reasons, all mythical. First of all, these are not very potent drugs. People tend to think that you can take a horse with a broken leg and make him insensible to pain through the use of these compounds. You can't. They are great for relieving minor aches and pains, but they will not keep a horse from limping if he really hurts.

"He must really be hurting. I gave him two bute and he's *still* limping."

Not at all. Just think of these drugs like you would think of any of the over-the-counter preparations that you buy for yourself. If you have a bit of a stiff back or a mild headache, aspirin and similar drugs can be very helpful in relieving pain. They will not, however, numb a serious problem, like a broken leg or torn tendon.

Other myths about these drugs abound. Flunixin meglumine is generally known as *the* drug for colic. In experimental models, the drug appears to be somewhat better than some of the other drugs in the same class at controlling the pain of colic, but it's not nearly as effective at controlling colic pain as other drugs from different classes.[7,8,9] Many trainers will tell you that phenylbutazone will make a horse "harder in the mouth" than the other drugs, but this seems to be an individual trainer bias rather than a consistent effect. Many trainers use phenylbutazone and don't have mouth problems.

How can you argue with someone who says that sort of thing, anyway? If someone says, "I think it does!" you can't exactly say, "No you don't."

Another effect of nonsteroidals is that they tend to inhibit the formation of blood clots. The dose required for this effect is smaller than that required for the relief of pain. Therefore, there are some medical conditions in which these drugs are used with that specific purpose in mind. Human heart-attack patients, for example, are frequently advised to take one aspirin per day to help "thin" the blood. While it really doesn't make the blood any thinner, it does help to decrease blood clotting, which is a big reason why heart attacks occur. In horses, in the treatment of laminitis, the prevention of clots may also be important. For this reason, as well as for pain relief, nonsteroidal anti-inflammatory drugs are among the most commonly prescribed for the treatment of this condition.[10]

While nonsteroidal drugs do have side effects, they are not very dangerous drugs. Everything has potential side effects if you abuse it. Take chocolate.

Here is a delicious, wonderful substance that is a perfect reward for a variety of occasions. After dinner, a small piece of chocolate is soothing and satisfying. Your mother loves you when you give her chocolate. But eat lots of chocolate and your teeth fall out and you get fat.

Nonsteroidal anti-inflammatory drugs are like that, too. Horse people have developed a great concern that these drugs are "hard on the kidneys" and cause stomach ulcers. *At the recommended doses, there has been no evidence of bad effects from these drugs.*

When you double the dose of a drug like bute, however, from two grams twice daily (a safe and frequently prescribed dose) to four grams twice daily, ulcers can occur. This is because the formation of prostaglandins, the same chemicals associated with pain production, is also important for the normal function of the cells of the stomach and intestines. If you overdose your horse with anti-prostaglandin drugs, you have the potential for causing ulcers. As for kidney problems, these occur very rarely, but they have been reported in the veterinary journals. Care should also be taken in giving bute to horses that are dehydrated.[11]

As with antibiotics, a bit of care should be taken in the use of these drugs with very young, old or sick horses. In all these animals, something about the kidney function may be different from that of a normal adult. In young animals, the kidney function is immature. In old animals, the ability of the kidneys to function may be drawing to a close. And in sick animals, kidney function may be depressed from the effects of disease. Nonsteroidal anti-inflammatory drug use should be watched closely in these animals.

One other thing: Since all of these drugs work in pretty much the same fashion, the bad side effects are cumulative, too. Don't assume that you can avoid trouble from an overdose of one drug by giving two or more in combination. Just follow the recommended dosage of these drugs and your horse should be fine.

TRANQUILIZERS

Tranquilizers are employed to help in the treatment of the horse because frequently, without them, a horse won't *allow* treatment. These are wonderful drugs that make working around horses much safer than it otherwise would be. They are very, very safe for the horse.

Acepromazine, one of the more commonly prescribed tranquilizers, is the only one with a significant side effect, and it's a rare one. In all male horses, acepromazine causes relaxation of the muscles of the penis. (For this reason, it's a great drug to use when you clean a horse's prepuce, or sheath.) Also, very, very occasionally, this drug can prevent a horse from bringing his penis back up into his sheath. This effect is usually temporary and is usually seen when high doses of the drug are given. Medical and even surgical treatment may be required if this happens. Fortunately, it almost never does.[12]

Tranquilizers are great drugs that temporarily induce tranquility. They will work, even for the most fractious animals, if you give them a large enough dose. When a horse resists being trailered, for example, a tranquilizer may help him overcome his anxiety about getting into that small moving box. Unfortunately, lessons learned under tranquilization may not be retained when the horse is fully alert.[13]

Calm horses are desirable, not only for medical reasons but also for riding reasons. Unfortunately, not every horse is calm, especially when some human hops up on his back and starts kicking him in the sides and sawing away at his mouth. When a horse shows a lack of tranquility because of odd human behavior, it is not a medical condition and it does not respond well to treatment. If you work a horse to make him tired before riding him, for example, you will find that the more you work him, the more energetic he is likely to get, as he gets into better and better shape. And some horses are just lunatics.

For those of you who show, giving your horse tranquilizers is a big "no-no." There are tests for these drugs, and horse show associations are not happy to find that competing horses have been tranquilized. Tranquilizing show horses is not a practice that you want to follow, unless you enjoy attending disciplinary hearings by your governing horse show body. As you might suspect, this has developed something of a closet industry for nontestable or natural tranquilizers. Unfortunately, if you own a horse that needs to be tranquilized, nothing natural has been shown to work.

If you peruse the shelves at feed stores or health food stores you will find a variety of substances that purport to be calming. Limited experience with this stuff in horses has shown little and inconsistent effects. Calcium, for instance, is known to calm people. Horses eat lots of calcium, in alfalfa hay, but extra calcium shouldn't do anything to or for your horse. The same with niacin, one of the B vitamins.

The amino acid tryptophane has also been touted as a natural tranquilizer. This is because tryptophane is a precursor for the formation of a chemical called serotonin. Serotonin is a chemical (a neurotransmitter) that occurs in the brain in high levels during sleep. Some say that the reason warm milk or a turkey dinner makes you so sleepy is that since these foods are high in tryptophane, they will secondarily cause higher levels of serotonin. Whether this works or not in horses (or people) is anybody's guess. High levels of tryptophane have been associated with liver problems in people, and for this reason the product is much more tightly controlled now than it was in years past.

Unfortunately, if your horse is the excitable type, no amount of training, riding or discipline is likely to solve the problem of excitability because the "problem" is most likely normal for that horse. With training and experience, many horses can be helped to overcome their fear of unfamiliar surroundings. Tranquilizers can be a temporary stopgap measure. But the best way to avoid having an excitable horse is not to buy one in the first place.

DIMETHYL SULFOXIDE—DMSO

One of the most frequently employed and interesting substances with which to treat horses is a chemical solvent. It has been credited with over thirty properties for the treatment of disease and is therefore used in a wide variety of applications in the horse. The substance goes by the name of dimethyl sulfoxide, mercifully abbreviated to DMSO.

DMSO is available in gel or liquid form. The liquid form can be given orally or intravenously (when diluted), or it can be applied on top of the skin; the gel is always used topically. The use of the drug is generally based on the veterinarian's experience. Fortunately, DMSO is a fairly benign substance. As frequently as it is used, surprisingly little study has gone into its application in horses.

As a therapeutic agent, DMSO is used primarily as an anti-inflammatory. There are a variety of ways that DMSO exerts its effect as an anti-inflammatory, the most important of which seems to be the neutralization of some of the destructive substances that are produced by the process of inflammation. In addition, DMSO has some of the same anti-inflammatory properties as do the steroids. DMSO can be used at the same time as these drugs. DMSO will even help protect tissues from injury induced by a lack of blood (called ischemia; you can make your finger ischemic by putting a tight rubber band around it, for instance).[14] There are a variety of other useful properties of DMSO, too. Because DMSO has such a wide array of alluring medical possibilities for treatment, it is used quite a bit in veterinary medicine.

DMSO is unique in that it can go through the skin and mucous membranes without disrupting them. Because of this property, it can be used as a carrier of other substances through the skin. When DMSO is mixed with corticosteroids, for example, the level of the corticosteroids in the tissue is increased by a factor of three! And because it can go through the skin, people who use DMSO report tasting it after they put it on (or in) their horse.

DMSO is very volatile. When it is absorbed through the skin, it rapidly enters the circulatory system. The DMSO travels around until it reaches the lungs, at which point it exits the system and gets breathed out. Of course, the air that is breathed out comes up the back of your mouth. That is why it can be tasted. People report that DMSO tastes like onions or garlic, but although the taste may be unpleasant it certainly isn't harmful. Application of DMSO without out gloves is generally not recommended right before an important date.

The wide variety of conditions that DMSO is used to treat almost defies belief. There are reports of using the stuff topically to treat swellings and systemically for muscle soreness; injecting it into joints; for disease of the nervous system; for treatment of colic and its associated effects; in the reproductive tract of the mare; for skin conditions; to accelerate wound healing; to prevent blood clotting and for laminitis, to name but a few. Because of its ability to penetrate membranes, DMSO is also commonly employed to help get drugs into areas that are hard to reach, like the brain or the chest cavity. So if it seems that your veterinarian is using DMSO to treat almost everything, it's because he or she probably is.

Disturbingly (and surprisingly) enough, there are no standard doses that have been generated for DMSO. For most drugs, dose ranges based on half-lives and desired blood levels have been established. With DMSO this is not the case. Furthermore, much of what DMSO is used for is outside the manufacturer's recommended uses. Finally, in the treatment of most medical conditions in the horse, no controlled studies have been done to establish how well it works in treating the conditions. In spite of all that isn't known about DMSO, its use seems to keep steaming right along.

Fortunately, considering how widely the stuff is used, DMSO is pretty benign and has a very low toxicity. Even though you can taste it if you get it on your skin, DMSO is really not at all dangerous, as some people would have you believe. It is so safe that you can drink it, and it can also be given intravenously (remember, it should be diluted first). Don't be surprised if DMSO gets suggested for the treatment of some condition in your horse. DMSO is not a wonder drug, nor is it a cureall, but it sure is interesting.[15]

"NONMEDICINE" REMEDIES

There are shelves fulls of nonmedicines for your horse in your local feed store. These products are all touted as having wonderful effects. Unfortunately, none of them have been tested to see if they do what they say they are going to do. None of them can really hurt your horse, however, since they generally contain proteins or vitamins. It's just that none of them have any evidence that they actually work, other than the testimonials of various pleased and satisfied people that you most likely don't know. Don't be surprised if your veterinarian is not a good source of information about these products. Understandably, your veterinarian will be somewhat reluctant to prescribe something when he or she has no idea at all if it will work. Since this sort of product seems to appear weekly, it's hard for a busy veterinarian to keep up with every new product that comes along. But you can try them. It depends on how you want to spend your money.

Many other drugs used in the treatment of the horse have not been mentioned here. These drugs have a variety of specific uses and are employed in the treatment of appropriate conditions. They should be used on the advice of your veterinarian.

No drug should be used indiscriminately. The most important thing to remember about the use of drugs is that they are generally safe and effective when used according to the directions. Problems begin when people deviate from the recommended doses or uses of certain substances. A number of factors are involved in the selection of a drug and drug dose such as the age of the horse, his physical condition and the type of problem being treated. Even the price of the drug itself can affect whether or not it is used (although a $150 drug that doesn't work isn't better than a $300 drug that does). The best source of information about horse drugs is—you guessed it—your veterinarian and not your trainer, farrier, mother-in-law or groom. So don't be afraid of using drugs in your horse. Just use them properly.

PART II

FEEDS AND FEEDING

4

What's in the Feed?

Horses need to be fed. They should be fed regularly. That being said, the myths begin.

An amazing amount of objective information about feeds and the feeding of horses exists. Scientific types have analyzed horse feed to its most minute components, fed varieties of combinations of these components to horses, fed diets lacking in some components to horses, studied, repeated studies and published the results (this is what scientists do for a living). Their results can be summed up and reported conclusively here. Adult horses need the following: hay or pasture for roughage, water (as much as they want) and possibly some access to salt and minerals.[1]

That's it.

Sure, there's a little bit more to feeding the horse than that. Otherwise, this would be a very short chapter. Young horses up to two years of age have different nutritional requirements than adults. But there's not much more to feeding *adult* horses than that. With feeds, remember the following acronym: KISS, which stands for "Keep It Simple, Silly." When someone says that you *have* to do this or you *can't* do that with regard to feeding, smile politely and then walk away. You're about to know better.

All feeds provide different amounts of the same things. All feeds contain energy, protein, vitamins and minerals. Anything else they provide, like ash and fiber and water, is basically filler that comes with the package. Feed is just fancy packaging for its component parts.

ENERGY

The most important component of feed is energy. Energy is the gasoline that runs the engine that is your horse. Energy provides the fuel to keep the heart beating, the lungs pumping and so forth. A certain amount of it is needed to keep things running—the level needed for maintenance—and more may be needed if you ask your horse to do strenuous things like jump fences, ford raging rivers or have babies. And you can be certain that if your horse is getting enough energy in his diet, he's getting enough of everything else, too. Energy is measured in calories (which is a measurement of heat produced when food is burned).

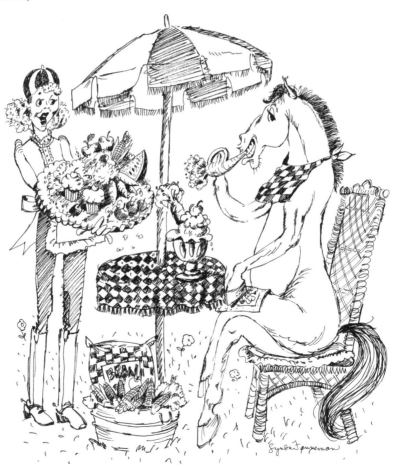

Feeding the adult horse.

Energy in feed comes from three sources: carbohydrates, fats and protein. Carbohydrates are easy to digest, supply lots of calories and are found in the highest levels in grains. Most of the energy in any diet comes from carbohydrates. Fats have even more energy than carbohydrates, two and a half times as much as the same amount of carbohydrate. Horse feed does not contain much fat, but fat is a good energy supplement for the horse.[2,3,4]

Proteins, the third potential source of energy in food, are the building blocks from which body tissue, enzymes and many hormones are made, and any extra protein beyond that which is required is used for energy. Protein, however, is not a good source of energy. It is hard for the body to digest, and it's the most expensive form of energy you can buy. Protein supplements cost a lot of money, and adult horses almost never need them. There is a lesson to be learned from this: *Don't overfeed protein.* You won't hurt the horse—feeding extra protein probably doesn't do anything except increase the amount of water the horse drinks (and the amount of urine he produces)—you'll just waste money.[5,6]

What does hard or easy to digest mean, anyway? Food is made up of a bunch of chemicals that are tied together by chemical bonds. In order for anything to be digested, these bonds have to be broken apart by the body, so that the chemicals can be absorbed and used by the body to keep the system operating. The ease with which these chemical bonds are broken down is what nutritionists mean by "hard" or "easy" to digest.

Carbohydrates are fairly simple chemical compounds, and the body breaks up their chemical bonds with ease and disdain. Complex chemical compounds, like proteins, are broken down slowly, and the body spends a good deal of digestive energy to harvest the energy that is available from them. The result is that there is less net energy available from protein than from carbohydrates or fats because so much energy is used by the body in getting the energy from the protein out of the feed. That's why overfeeding protein is wasteful, expensive and dumb.

VITAMINS, MINERALS AND OTHER FEED COMPONENTS

"Vitamin" is a broad term used to describe a number of unrelated organic substances that occur in many foods in small amounts. These are generally used by the body to help run the chemical reactions that go on as part of everyday living.[7] It's pretty difficult to make a horse's diet deficient in vitamins.

Minerals are also useful in many of the chemical reactions of the body. Some minerals are essential components of amino acids (the building blocks of proteins), hormones and vitamins. They also are important in some of the body's tissues (for instance, bone needs calcium).[8]

The rest of what makes up feed, like ash and fiber, is basically garbage. Ash is the residue you get when you burn feed during analysis. Fiber is fairly inert matter that is most obvious in the stems of the hay your horse eats. Neither has much nutritional value. Ash and fiber are like the cardboard box that your breakfast cereal comes in, without the good reading material. You can't get horse feed without the ash and fiber.[9]

WATER

Water is necessary for all normal body functions. While water has no nutritional value, it is absolutely essential for life. The horse must restore the liquids that his body loses during the day, through breathing, sweating and eliminating waste products. Feed is a poor source of water, as you might imagine, since most horse feed is dried prior to feeding, so horses need to have unlimited access to all the water they want. Water should always be clean and fresh.

You're probably reading this thinking, "My horse gets a scientifically balanced formula of four grains with specific supplements added for coat, tail and hoof. What does all this have to do with anything, anyway?" Keep reading. Remember the "horses are like cars" analogy (from the Preface). You probably own a car (unless you own too many horses). Your car needs gas, oil and regular maintenance. Your horse needs enough feed to supply his energy and protein needs, and he also needs water. The rest is all fuzzy dice and little dolls that have bobbing heads. (Never act like one of those dolls when someone tells you something that you *have* to do, by the way.)

Since all feeds are packages containing varying amounts of the same things, it's not that one feed is better than another, it's that each feed is *different* from another. The differences make certain feeds more appropriate for some situations than others. For example, alfalfa hay has more calcium, more energy (from all sources) and more protein than grass-type hays. All hays have less energy than grains. Most grains have less protein in them than hays.

So if your horse is too fat (as many are) you should choose a feed that has less energy in it. A grass type of hay, for example, may be more suitable for your overweight horse than a higher-energy hay like alfalfa. The grass hay isn't better, it's just more appropriate. A high-energy feed, like a grain, would probably not be a great thing to feed him, either. See how easy this is? Keep It Simple, Silly.

This book cannot analyze all types of feed. Endless tables on this sort of thing, produced by animal nutritionists, are available and absolutely mindnumbing to read. They are informative, however. If you want to know all the particulars about a certain feed, look them up in nutrition books. Then go on to the next chapters to read about how (and how not) to apply the feeds that are available to your horse.

5

Feeding the Adult Horse

Now that you have the basics of feed components down, it's time for a few rules of thumb—guidelines for you to feed your adult horse.

Rule #1—The majority of your horse's diet must be made up of hay or hay products. That's the way it is.[1]

Rule #2—To maintain your horse's weight, feed him, on the average, 1.5 to 2 percent of his body weight per day in dry feed. That is, if your horse weighs a thousand pounds, he will need, on the average, fifteen to twenty pounds of dry feed per day to keep his weight up and his heart beating and so forth. Some horses need more than this, and some horses seem to live on air.

Rule #3—Your horse's weight is about right when you can feel his ribs easily but not see them. Most show horses are fat. Fat is apparently pleasing to the owners of horses in the show ring, although the horses are not able to express their opinions on the matter. Horses, like people, can exist at a wide variety of weight levels. Also, like people, they will generally happily eat at every opportunity. It's one of the things that horses like to do the most. (In the wild, horses spend 50 to 60 percent of their time eating.) Therefore, it's usually easy to have a fat horse—but remember that fat is no more healthy for the horse than for the owner. (If you want to have an idea of what condition your horse is in, refer to the table of individual condition scores in the Notes section at the end of the book.)[2]

On the other hand, the principal cause of skinny horses is not enough feed. If anyone asks you why his or her horse is too thin, you'll generally be right if you say, "He's probably not getting enough to eat." More on this later.

Rule #4—The more work your horse does, the more energy he needs. That is, the more work he does, the more feed he needs, since energy comes from the feed, right?

Work can be described as light, medium or heavy. Light work occurs at the trot and canter. Medium work causes the horse to sweat. Heavy work causes the horse to lather and breathe heavily. For light work, the horse may need an extra three to five pounds of feed per hour of work. For medium work, the horse may need an additional five to eight pounds of feed per hour of work. For heavy work, the horse may need an extra eight to twelve pounds of feed per hour of work.[3] Another way to look at this is that light, medium or heavy work can increase the energy requirements for your horse by 25, 50 or 100 percent respectively.[4]

"Wait a second," you say, "if I'm working my horse hard he may need a whole lot of extra feed. That's going to cost a lot of extra money."

That's right, it's going to cost extra money to work your horse hard. But there are no real options here. If you work your horse hard and don't give him extra feed, he will use energy stored up in his body. Keep it up and your horse will be exhausted and very skinny.

A little arithmetic will indicate that if you work your thousand-pound horse hard for two hours every day (hopefully you don't), he may need up to forty-four pounds of feed a day. There is no way that you will be able to get forty-four pounds of hay into your horse. You just can't. Forty-four pounds of hay won't fit into his stomach. This is referred to as a diet being bulk limited. Therefore, if your horse needs extra energy, you have to give him something else.

Rule #5—If your horse exercises and needs extra energy, give it to him. He does not need extra protein, vitamins or minerals because of exercise.[5] He needs extra energy. There are two good sources: grain and fat.

Grain is a great source of energy. Corn, for example, is used with up to 90 percent efficiency by the horse. That is, of all the energy in a pound of corn (measured by burning the corn), 90 percent of it is available for use by the horse's body. Even the best hay is only about 55 percent digestible. A lot of energy fits into a small amount of grain.[6]

With fats, you can get even more energy. On an equal weight basis, fats have two and a half times more energy than grains. Corn oil is a readily available and very palatable source of fat that you can get at the grocery store. Experimentally, diets with up to 12 percent fat have been fed to horses with no problems. By increasing the fat content of your horse's diet, you can increase the amount of energy in the diet without increasing the volume of feed that he has to digest.[7]

GRAINS

Grains are a rich source of myths for horse owners. For some reason, grains are sometimes assailed as a dangerous feed for horses, capable of causing all sorts of dietary and metabolic ills, like laminitis. Of course, improperly handled your vacuum cleaner could probably do some harm, too. The other reason that people try not to feed grain to their horses is because people are afraid that they will lose control of their normally docile friends, that they will become "high" and unmanageable and crazy and wild.

Grains are merely concentrated energy sources. If you feed your horse lots of energy and if you exercise him regularly, there is a good chance that he will be energetic. That's the point. If you ask for lots of energy *from* your horse, you have to give lots of energy *to* your horse.

The fear that feeding grains to horses will make them high is not something that has been researched, however. No one has ever looked at horses that are being fed grains and then made an effort to record if they become unmanageable as a result. The point is, if you want your horse to have a lot of energy and not get terribly thin, you have to feed him a concentrated energy source.

Remember, the harder your horse works, the better he will feel. If you work your horse and feed him properly he is going to feel great and full of energy. There is a term for this. The term is "normal."

Grain doesn't "make horses high." It is a source of energy. In association with regular exercise, a good diet makes horses feel good. There's really no way around this.

Of all the grains, corn is the worst, right? Corn will make them really high, right? Well, no. Corn is the most efficiently digested of feeds. If you give a horse one pound of corn, he will get almost twice as much energy from it than he will from a pound of oats. Comparing corn to other grains is like comparing apples to oranges. You need to feed *less* corn to get the same amount of energy that you get from a larger amount of oats. It's actually less expensive to feed corn than it is to feed any of the other grains.[6]

Corn is also supposed to be a "hot" feed. What this myth refers to really isn't clear. Corn certainly doesn't make horses sweat. Perhaps people have tried to feed the same amounts of corn as they do lesser-energy grains like oats and concluded that the horses get more energetic when fed corn, making corn "hotter" than oats. This is true, and it is also what makes corn a good, economical source of energy. A mixture of corn and alfalfa doesn't have any greater "heating" effect than does a mixture of oats and timothy grass hay.[8]

That's not to say that grain is absolutely benign. You can overfeed grain, of course. Small amounts of extra grain over a long period of time cause obesity. Large amounts of grain over a short period of time are associated with a condition called laminitis, or founder, a very serious condition that can cause dramatic and devastating consequences for your horse's feet. If you suspect that your horse has eaten a large amount of grain in the past couple of hours, call your veterinarian and have your horse treated right away. This is a real emergency. If you can prevent the development of laminitis you're much better off than if you're trying to fix what has already occurred ("An ounce of prevention …").

Most grains that are fed to horses have been processed. By cracking, crimping or flaking the kernel of the grain, the surface area for digestion is supposedly increased and feed efficiency is improved. Right?

Well, maybe not. Crimping oats has been shown to increase their digestibility by only about 5 percent.[9] Furthermore, even such dramatic steps as the cutting and vacuum cleaning of oats does not affect their digestibility.[10] Processed grains are not worth a premium price.

If your horse requires more energy, for whatever reason, grains are a great source. It probably doesn't matter what kind of grain you use and if it's been processed. Don't feed too much.

WHEN TO FEED

Ah, but when to feed this energy? Believe it or not, there is virtually no research on the best time to give energy to your horse that is exercising. Most horses—show, trail or pleasure—never exercise at anything near maximum capacity, so the time you feed extra energy to these horses is not critical. These horses just need regular feeding, according to their condition.

When to feed becomes particularly interesting, however, when applied to horses that are pushed to maximum exercise levels, such as endurance horses or racehorses. It is well known that glucose (sugar) solutions given orally rapidly show up in the horse's bloodstream (the glucose in grain is rapidly taken up, too). Interestingly enough, however, most of the glucose in the blood is not immediately used by the body during exercise. Rather, it goes to help build up the body's energy stores in the muscle.[7] So it's not likely that anything that you feed your horse immediately before exercise is going to make any difference in his performance, at least in the couple of hours immediately after eating.

In fact, there is some evidence that a lot of feed prior to exercise may be detrimental to performance. A rise in glucose in the blood is followed by a rise in insulin. Insulin helps get the glucose into the cells of the body, but by doing so it results in a *decrease* in the glucose in the blood. In human athletes, eating an hour before exercise may actually cause a more rapid onset of exhaustion due to this effect (although this has been disputed by some researchers).[11,12] There is some thought that this same effect may also be seen in horses. Feed also adds weight to the horse's abdomen that may slow him down when he exercises.[7] So there are recommendations made that horses be fasted on the day of an event, to avoid these effects.[3]

After all that, this next bit is going to make you crazy. There is also evidence that eating during exercise is of benefit to human athletes in events lasting more than two hours.[11] The extra blood glucose gained from eating seems to provide increased endurance in these athletes.

So what do you do with your horse during exercise? Well, if you extrapolate the data from human and horse sources, you might reasonably come up with the following conclusions:

1. The best way to have a healthy, energetic horse is to exercise him regularly and feed him well.
2. For exercise where quick energy is required, feeding prior to a race is probably of no benefit and possibly detrimental.
3. Where endurance is desired, feeding during a race may be helpful. (There is no evidence to show that this will cause intestinal discomfort, either.)
4. Most show horses are too fat. They don't exercise hard enough to make how you feed them that important anyway.
5. More research needs to be done.
6. Anybody who claims to have all the answers is an idiot.

HAY

How about hay myths? Alfalfa hay takes a real beating around the barns. Alfalfa is bad, right? Alfalfa is hard on the horse's kidneys, right? (You just know it because horses tend to urinate more when fed alfalfa than when on other feeds.) Wrong.

Alfalfa hay is a good feed source for horses. Alfalfa has been around only since about 500 B.C.[9] You'd think that if it were all that bad, someone would have noticed by now, wouldn't you? In some areas, alfalfa is the cheapest and most readily available hay. It has much more protein in it than horses need. It has a higher calcium level than other hays and grains. Horses like it.

It's the protein in alfalfa hay that makes the horses urinate so much. Protein has a lot of nitrogen in it, and nitrogen is filtered from the blood by the kidneys. It's one of the things that kidneys do. Removing the nitrogen doesn't wear the kidneys out any more than brushing your teeth wears your teeth out. As a matter of fact, it has been suggested that the increased kidney activity might be *beneficial* to the horse by allowing more active removal of body toxins.[9] If you give a horse lots of protein, expect urine, ammonia and wet stalls. Don't expect the kidneys to give out.

PROCESSED FEEDS

Hay, like all feed products, can be processed and packaged. It can be chopped up and mixed with molasses, chopped and steamed into cubes or bound into little pellets. Well, what about processed hay? Is it bad?

On the plus side, processed hay (and pellets) is easy to store, easy to measure and eaten with virtually no waste. However, even though the hay is chopped up, it is not more efficiently digested than loose hay.[9] On the minus side, horses are able to eat processed hay more quickly than loose hay and probably don't have as much fun eating it. As a result they may tend to get bored and develop fun habits like cribbing and weaving in the stall. It is commonly thought that there is a higher incidence of processed hay products getting stuck in the esophagus and causing choke, although there's no data to support such a belief (not that that has ever kept anyone from believing something).

And of course, with processed hays, you don't know what kind of hay went into the manufacturing process. But cubes and pellets are certainly not waste dumps for bad hay, as is sometimes alleged. Feed manufacturers would not stay in business making a product that was detrimental to your horse's health. There's really nothing inherently wrong with these products.

There are also a variety of processed-grain products on the market. They look like dog food. Horses eat these products just fine, and there's nothing wrong with them. It's just that there's no reason to think that they're better than any other horse feed. Since they are processed and packaged and advertised, you can be sure that they will be more expensive than plain old homely grains. You cannot be sure that they are any better for your horse.

VITAMINS

Vitamins make up a huge portion of every feed store, and no packaged grain ration would be complete without the "proper" vitamins. Fortunately, it's quite difficult to hurt horses by giving them vitamins (unless you are just dead set on giving dramatic overdoses of these otherwise benign substances). But horses generally don't need extra vitamins in their diet.

Horses obtain vitamins in their bodies from the bacteria that are in their intestines. Horse feeds are also a rich source of vitamins. Without question, vitamins are very important for the chemical reactions of the body. However, it is virtually impossible to make a horse vitamin deficient as long as you feed him. The requirements for vitamins do not go up during exercise, either, except possibly, and slightly, those for vitamin B_{12}.[5] Horses synthesize all of the vitamins that they need. People don't. People need B vitamins from their diet and vitamin C, too. Not horses. They can make their own.

It's fairly common practice to give horses, especially race horses, a jug of fluids and vitamins prior to a competition. It's supposed to help them run faster. There's no reason to believe it should.

Nutritionists are divided about the need for vitamin supplements in people. The thing is, people tend to eat such poor diets that vitamin supplements can be helpful in some cases. People were not meant to exist on potato chips and soft drinks. Horses were meant to exist on grass and water. They are well equipped to do just that.

MINERALS

It's even harder to make a horse diet that's deficient in minerals. Horses love to eat dirt and lick barns. Their feed is just loaded with minerals, too. If you supply your horse with a salt block that contains trace minerals, he will never have a problem with a mineral deficiency.

Horses do not eat anything because they feel that they are mineral deficient. People will tell you, "Horses eat dirt because they are deficient in minerals," or because "something is lacking in their diet." Horses don't know or sense that anything is missing in their diet, even if it is.

It has been well demonstrated that animals do not eat vitamins or minerals (or anything else) according to what they need, with the single exception of sodium, which is one of the components of salt.[14] Your horse will not become sodium deficient if you give him *anything* to eat. Allowed to consume vitamins and minerals in unlimited amounts, horses will eat different amounts according to how they like the taste.

There is absolutely no relationship between dietary mineral levels and consumption of dirt, rocks, manure or wood.[3,15,16,17,18] When ponies are fed diets that are lacking in calcium, they do not develop a liking for calcium-containing supplements.[19] Most likely, horses eat dirt and that kind of stuff because they are bored.[9]

Horses break into carrot bags all the time, but there have never been any reports of carrot deficiencies in horses.

The eating of stuff that horses don't normally eat is called pica. Not only does this not reflect a "deficiency," but it's usually harmless, unless the horse eats a lot of sand or some weird foreign substance, like the rubber fencing that was so popular several years ago.

Horses also love to eat manure. That certainly isn't harmful, either (although it is a way that parasites are transmitted). Manure is relatively nutritious. You can *make* your horse eat manure if you starve him or feed him diets that don't have fiber or protein in them,[20] but why would you keep a horse and not feed him something with fiber and protein (like hay)?

Of course, when your horse eats manure it certainly is gross. You feel like he is somehow socially retarded. Horses will eat anything that isn't moving, and eating manure gives them something else to do to make you tear your hair.

ELECTROLYTES

Electrolytes (a chemical term that defining wouldn't help or even be interesting) are salts. Horses generally don't need extra electrolytes. Even in the hottest weather, horses get all the electrolytes that they need in their feed. Feed is loaded with salts. People used to take electrolytes prior to exercise in the form of salt pills. What nutritionists found was that this caused people to retain water and not sweat well, which is dangerous in hot weather. Electrolyte supplementation is usually not needed in normal working horses.

It is possible to make a horse sweat out a significant portion of his electrolytes by riding him hard in hot weather and not stopping to rest him or to give him water. During a hundred-mile endurance ride, for example, it's probably a good idea to give your horse extra electrolytes along with lots of water. Indeed, providing water, glucose and electrolytes to working endurance horses does seem to delay fatigue.[21,22]

If you exhaust your horse, it is possible that he will be depleted of water and electrolytes. When horses exercise, they lose water much faster than electrolytes. No matter how much salt you give your horse in hot weather, if you don't let him have water, you're going to be in big trouble. Electrolyte depletion causes all sorts of bizarre signs, like weakness, staggering or an interesting condition where the diaphragm contracts in rhythm with the heart. This is called thumps (or synchronous diaphragmatic flutter, if you must know).[23,24] Ideally, you are sensitive enough to recognize that your horse is getting tired long before it gets to the point of electrolyte depletion.

THE OVERWEIGHT HORSE

If a horse gets too fat, it's your fault. After all, horses love to eat and they can only eat what you feed them. Horses eat continuously in the wild and generally don't get fat, but they also walk around all day long and eat low-calorie grass, as opposed to things like alfalfa and bags of horse treats. A horse in the stall can't get the exercise that is required to keep from getting fat if he's fed too much. Fat horses are not able to tolerate exercise as well as horses in good condition. Fat acts as a layer of insulation all around them. Being so well insulated, fat horses have trouble getting rid of the heat that exercise generates; they can overheat and stop working. In addition, chronic obesity is definitely associated with laminitis and with the occurrence of fat tumors (lipomas) in the abdomen. Lipomas can twist around the intestine and result in your horse going to the hospital for colic surgery.[20]

Don't let your horse get overweight. If he does, reduce his feed or, preferably, feed him a lower-calorie hay so that he'll still have something to eat (and to help pass the time). And exercise him, too.

THE UNDERWEIGHT HORSE

A thin horse, on the other hand, can be a much more involved diagnostic problem, although most of the time it isn't. A whole lot of things can result in a horse being underweight, but as a practical matter the most common cause of thinness has to do with feed. Generally, either the feed is of poor quality and incapable of supplying his nutritional needs or the amount of feed supplied is insufficient for the energy demands made of him.

Some huge majority of underweight horses are underfed. Finding out that your horse is skinny because he's not getting enough to eat is like finding out that the washing machine doesn't work because it wasn't plugged in. You're glad to find out what the cause is, but you feel kind of stupid all the same and you probably really wish it had been something else. With horses and weight loss, the obvious thing (not enough feed) is the most common cause of the problem and the first thing you should look for if your horse is too thin.

For instance, if your skinny horse is in a pasture with three fat horses, he may indeed have a problem with his kidneys or his liver or his teeth. These problems are the types of things that most people like to look for and are the first things that they think about. They're not obvious. Generally, however, this problem is related to herd dominance. If your horse is the only one in the herd that's too thin, he is most likely not getting enough to eat because he's the lowest on the totem pole. While it makes sense to investigate other causes of weight loss in this situation, it makes the most sense to address the most obvious potential problem first and feed the horse separately or place a number of piles of feed at distances from each other that help reduce the effects of the dominant behavior of the other horses on your skinny horse.

If your horse that lives in a stall doesn't weigh enough, you *should* get his teeth checked and make sure that he's been dewormed, but make sure that he's getting fed enough, too. Although poor teeth are reported to be a cause of slow or inefficient eating habits, they are rarely bad enough to keep a horse from eating and are, in the author's experience, an extremely uncommon cause of weight loss. Horses in stables have a minimal exposure to internal parasites— their manure gets cleaned out regularly and they usually don't get exposed to other horse manure—so parasites are unlikely to be a significant cause of weight loss in stabled horses. Check for them, sure, but expect to find the problem elsewhere.

In stabled situations you will assume that your horse is getting enough feed, but since you never actually distribute the food yourself you don't really know how much he's getting. Even if you ask for extra feed, it doesn't mean that your horse is getting it (this is not to impugn anyone's credibility, but you do have to investigate all of the possibilities). Also make sure that you evaluate the exercise level required of your horse and be sure he is getting enough energy to provide what he is asked to spend.

It is also possible you have a horse that doesn't put on weight easily. You have friends like that and you hate them, too. There are metabolic differences in certain body types. For horses that don't like to put on weight, the only solution is to give them more feed than you think they are likely to need. Feeding these horses more calories in a smaller package, such as what is provided in grains and fats, will help keep weight on horses that tend to be thin.

Some horses have weird metabolic conditions or infections or something else that makes them too thin. But these horses are in the minority of those that don't weigh enough. Look into other causes for weight loss in the thin horse *after* you have evaluated his diet and particularly if he does not respond to dietary changes.

Also, realize that it is going to take time for your horse to gain weight if he is too thin. Even if you successfully identify undernutrition as a cause of weight loss, you have to be patient while your horse is putting the weight back on; horses can't gain a hundred pounds overnight. It can take months to get an underweight horse back to where you want him. If you need some sort of reassurance that your horse is putting on weight, a weight tape (they are available at most feed stores) will help you measure the gains (and hopefully increase your patience).

WATER

One little note about water. Water, as you know, is absolutely critical for your horse's existence. That your horse should have access to fresh water is obvious. If you think that your horse isn't drinking enough water while at home, make sure the water supply is clean. Also make sure that something isn't wrong with the watering system (for example, horses can receive electric shocks from certain types of malfunctioning waterers, which renders them, understandably, somewhat reluctant to risk taking a drink).

Sometimes horses won't drink water at horse shows; the water there may taste different. If your horse tends not to drink while at horse shows, you may want to "doctor" his water supply. At home, you can add things to his water, like sugar or salt or vinegar or peppermint (horses especially like sweet tastes), to flavor it. Then, when at a new stabling facility, add the same substance to the water and disguise any funny taste that the different water may have and give it a known funny taste. Fortunately, most horses don't have this problem.[25]

All this nutrition stuff can be summed up rather succinctly. Your adult horse does need roughage. He will need extra energy if you work him hard. He does not need extra vitamins or minerals. In the specific circumstance of hours of hard work in hot weather he may need some extra electrolytes. He needs lots of water. Everything else is like the fuzzy dice that hang from your rearview mirror.

6

Youth, Pregnancy and Other Stresses

At times, a horse may have requirements for some nutrients that are quite different from those needed to maintain body weight or for exercise. Growing horses, pregnant mares, lactating mares and even older horses have slightly different problems and nutritional requirements than mature adult horses. It is very important to keep these in mind so you can properly feed your horse. Still, this is pretty simple stuff and you shouldn't make yourself crazy trying to do the right thing.

Most of the differences between feeding normal adult horses and those requiring extra stuff have to do with the amount of energy that is needed. Most horses, when they find themselves in a situation where they need an extra "something," need additional energy. Specific examples follow.

GROWING UP

The most important thing to keep in mind about your growing young horse is that his or her diet must be balanced. In a balanced diet, not only are all of the nutrients supplied in the proper amounts, they are supplied in the proper amounts relative to each other. It's not particularly difficult to keep a ration balanced. Feed tables provide the information you need to calculate this sort of thing if you are so inclined.[1]

BABIES

Initially, of course, growing babies get all of their nutritional needs from their mother's milk and, happily, you really don't have to do anything except feed the mare to make sure that the baby is getting all it needs in its first few weeks. In a fairly short period of time, though, foals will begin to look around and notice that mom is eating hay and grain. Being curious sorts, they will figure that if Mom's eating the stuff, then they might as well try it out, too. Pretty soon, Mom and baby will be eating beside each other, providing a wide variety of warm photographic opportunities.

It is often desirable to give these babies supplemental feed of their own. The baby horse is growing. Growing requires a whole bunch of energy. (Those of you with teenagers will appreciate how hard it is to keep your refrigerator full.) If a mare doesn't produce a lot of milk or has some sort of disease that prevents her from producing much milk (both conditions are pretty rare), there is a possibility that she may not be giving her foal enough energy or nutrients. Also, after the foal reaches three months of age, it can probably not get enough nutrition from milk alone anyway. Therefore, one of the easiest ways to give your growing foal extra nutrition is to provide a creep feeder.

The creep feeder is a clever device that allows the baby to eat his feed but prevents Mom from doing so, generally by having an opening in the feeder that is too small to allow the exasperated mare to get her nose in. The creep feeder should be in an obvious place, like near the waterer or any other place that the mare likes to hang out, so the baby will begin to notice that it is there. Eventually he'll begin to investigate what's in "that thing by the waterer," and he'll begin munching away in no time at all.

Feed should be given to the foal every day, in quantities so that he can have feed any time he wants it. One of the big advantages of creep feeding is that it gets the baby used to eating on his own. It has been shown that foals that have been given creep feed several weeks prior to weaning tend to eat better once they are weaned and are also less susceptible to the stress of weaning. There's nothing worse than having a baby say, "Okay, take me from my Mom and I'll just starve." The foal should have his own creep feed preparation and not just the same grain that the mare gets. Foals have a higher need for certain nutrients in relation to the amount of energy than do their mothers. There are a number of good creep feeder mixes available.[1]

The feed for a young foal should be balanced for minerals. Horse diets frequently tend to be high in calcium with respect to phosphorus, due, at least in part, to the high calcium content in the alfalfa hay many horses are fed. This imbalance can be adjusted, generally by providing additional phosphorus in the diet. An imbalance of calcium and phosphorus is only one of a number of

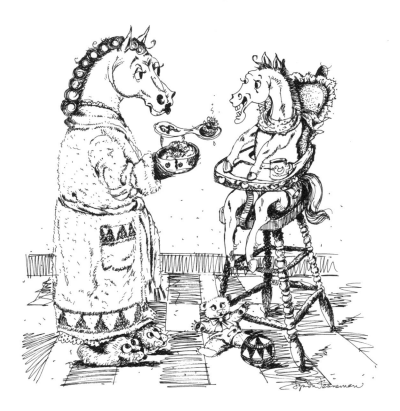

Feeding the baby horse.

factors that have been associated with a whole host of problems broadly referred to as "developmental orthopedic disease" and seen in specific problems such as contracted tendons, osteochondrosis (a developmental disease of the joint cartilage) and epiphysitis (a developmental disease of the areas that the bones grow from), to name a few.[2,3,4] Some veterinarians recommend feeding additional copper, beyond that which is recommended by the National Research Council, to young horses as a way to help avoid some of these problems.[5,6]

The best way to help prevent developmental problems is to use balanced feed products to feed your baby and, indeed, to all growing young horses. What needs to be done for *your* growing horse is influenced by his diet and the area where you live. When desired, feed can be analyzed to see what's in it. If necessary, the feed can then be supplemented to provide the proper balance of minerals. Your veterinarian can (and should) help you with this.

WEANLINGS

The ideal time for weaning is open to discussion, and the "best" time is probably the one that works out best for your schedule, since it will undoubtedly be a horrible inconvenience to the mare and foal whenever you choose to do it. Left on their own in the wild, mares usually don't wean their babies until one or two years of age! Foals have been weaned as early as two months, and although there is some evidence to show that early weaned foals actually grow better than those that are weaned later,[7] you really have to watch the diets of early weaned babies closely. They can't live on just hay and water.

Whenever you decide to wean your baby, be prepared for a whole lot of screaming from the mare and foal. The best way to wean is to separate the two of them as far from each other as possible and try not to pay too much heed to the resultant cries of anguish.

There is a great deal of concern about making weanlings grow too fast. Possibly too much concern. High levels of carbohydrate intake in the young horse have been associated with a variety of the developmental orthopedic disease conditions mentioned previously.[8,9,10,11] Unfortunately, for those of you who like black and white answers, some other studies have failed to show any orthopedic problems in rapidly growing foals.[12,13,14] However, it is often recommended that extremely rapid growth rates or growth spurts (caused by inconsistent levels of nutrition) be avoided in weanling horses.[3]

Since people generally worry about too rapid growth in their young horses, sometimes they overreact and end up starving them. Protein and energy are the two major nutrient factors that affect the growth of young horses.[1] If you restrict either the amount of energy or the amount of protein that the growing horse gets, you can very effectively limit his growth and end up with a much smaller horse than you had anticipated. Although a horse with developmental orthopedic problems is not desirable, neither is one that is rough-coated and stunted.[4]

The point of all this is that the problem of developmental orthopedic disease is very complex and there are no easy answers as to how to prevent or treat the condition. Not feeding one thing or overfeeding another is not the only answer to a problem that has nutritional, hormonal and hereditary influences.[15] While rations should be inspected and adjusted for obvious abnormalities, a well-balanced diet for growth should not contribute to bone abnormalities, even when the foals are allowed unlimited access to the feed.[4,16]

In spite of all of the confusion and controversy regarding developmental orthopedic problems, there are some general recommendations that can be made. The ideal growth rate for young horses has not been established, so it's impossible to tell you exactly what your weanling needs to be fed on, say, day 187 of life. Young animals have to be fed as individuals. Here are some specific suggestions:

1. Weanlings can and should have free access to hay. They can't overeat hay, and it's good for them.
2. They should also be supplemented with a balanced grain mix containing at least 14 percent protein.[1] "Balanced" means with respect to vitamins, minerals and so forth.
3. No more than 60 percent of the weanling's ration should be in the form of grain.[3]
4. Weanlings may eat from 2 to 3.5 percent of their body weight per day in dry feed. A three-hundred-pound yearling may therefore eat up to 10.5 pounds of feed (hay and grain) a day.[1]

UP TO TWO YEARS

The older the young horse gets, the closer his requirements get to that of an adult. The percentage of feed that he eats, compared to his body weight, decreases with age, and the proportion of hay that makes up his diet should increase. By the time the horse reaches one year of age, the ratio of hay to grain should be no more than 50:50.[3] These horses should always have ready access to hay and, of course, always be fed a diet that is balanced. Many of the developmental problems will have shown up by one year of age and if your baby has made it this far, things will probably be all right.

GESTATION

Until the last three months of pregnancy, mares don't need any nutrition beyond what you would give them anyway.[1] That is, the nutritional requirements of a mare do not change at all during the first eight months that they are pregnant. They don't need extra anything. Don't give them extra anything, either, because you can make your mare too fat and funny looking. It's not healthy.

It is not true, however, that fat mares have problems getting pregnant. They don't, and they have an easier time of it than skinny mares.[17] It's still not healthy for them.

During the last three months, however, energy and protein requirements do increase. Not dramatically, mind you, but they do go up a little bit. Energy requirements are estimated to go up by 11, 13 and 20 percent during the ninth, tenth and eleventh months of gestation, respectively (the gestation period is about eleven months). You add this to the rest of the mare's regular ration. If you feed the extra energy in a grain ration that supplies from 14 to 18 percent protein, this should be about all that is necessary to provide the extra energy and protein needed for the growing baby and to get your mare ready to make milk.[18, 19]

LACTATION

Making milk requires a lot of energy from the mare. Because of this, her feed requirements will increase, especially early in lactation, when the baby seems to be hanging on to the udder all the time (and probably is). A mare in early lactation may eat up to 3 percent of her body weight per day in feed, which can be up to twice as much as she may need to maintain herself without the baby.[1]

You will most likely have to supplement the mare with some grain to help her maintain her weight while she is making milk. A variety of products are available for this. The mare's protein requirement goes up slightly with milk production, so the grain ration should probably be a bit higher in protein than that which you would feed regularly.

It is interesting that what you feed the mare doesn't really seem to affect the composition of the milk. There haven't been many studies on this, but it appears that lactating mares fed hay and grain produce milk of the same nutritional caliber as do lactating mares fed just hay.[1] As long as you realize that your mare is going to need extra nutrition when she makes milk, she will continue to do so. You can't make her produce "better" milk through the feed.

OLD HORSES

The biggest problem with older horses is that they experience a decline in the efficiency with which they digest their feed.[20] There's nothing you can do to reverse this process. You also have to make sure that your older horse is being cared for in such a way as to obtain the maximum efficiency from what he gets. Such things as proper tooth care and parasite control are very important in older horses. So is proper nutrition.

In spite of their decline in digestive efficiency (and in spite of what you might have heard), old horses generally do *not* need special diets. However, if your old horse is losing weight and there is no obvious or serious cause (like a kidney or liver problem), you should try to either increase his amount of feed, increase the amount of energy in his feed by adding grain or fat, or do both. Also, as horses age they can begin to lose teeth, making it hard for them to eat anything. These horses can do very well if fed a slop made of pelleted feeds soaked in water.[21]

The nutritional needs of horses change during the course of their lives.[22] Depending on how old a horse is or what he is doing at the time, certain dietary requirements may increase. These increases are always in the need for energy and occasionally in the need for protein.

No specific product is the "best" for your horse, just as no specific car is the best to get you down the highway (although, like feeds, some cars are much more expensive than others). In order to do the best job in satisfying your horse's particular needs, you have to keep his requirements in mind and make sure that you give a proper, balanced ration, particularly to growing horses. If you can do that, you will go a long way toward ensuring that you have a healthy horse to enjoy.

PART III

ROUTINE CARE

7

Vaccinations

The "horses are like cars" analogy keeps coming up. Preventive maintenance for your horse is like making sure that oil in your car gets changed. If you don't do it as scheduled, pretty soon it will catch up with you.

Preventive care involves a few straightforward things. Feed and water, for instance, prevent a lot of problems, such as lethargy and weight loss and, eventually, death.

Other things that you should do regularly to maintain your horse's health are less obvious but only slightly less important. This chapter will try to separate the facts from the fiction about the vaccines available for your horse. Other important subjects, like dewormers and care of the teeth, will be discussed later.

"Horses need to be vaccinated _____ times per year." Anyone who tells you that there is a right answer to the question isn't giving you a full understanding of the vaccine world. It would be wonderful (and much easier) if there were a clearly defined "right" vaccination program. But, with vaccination, as in most of life, circumstances dictate how things are done. How often you vaccinate your horse depends.

Why vaccinate horses at all? Horses are vaccinated to help protect them from nasty things that live in their world, like viruses or bacterial toxins. In his natural and unvaccinated state a horse exposed to these things may get sick.

HOW VACCINATIONS WORK

There are many things the body does when it is sick. One of the most important responses is the creation of antibodies. Antibodies are made by the body's immune system, the system that helps protect the body from the bad things in the outside world. The immune system allows the body to distinguish foreign substances from itself and then to neutralize, eliminate and metabolize those foreign substances.[1] Antibodies are produced to help the body get rid of whatever invader happens to be visiting at the time.

When the body is first exposed to one of these invaders, antibodies are produced slowly. Eventually, some antibody level (titer) against the specific invader is reached. The antibodies are produced in reaction to a specific part of the offending intruder, called the antigen. Happily, the second time the intruder (and its antigen) is seen by the body, the immune system is able to produce antibodies at very high levels very rapidly. This is called an anamnestic response (it is to learn words like this that medical schools were created). High antibody levels assist the body in getting rid of the invader.

In the process of fighting off disease, the production of antibodies is part of the natural response to eliminating the offending agent. Veterinarians are able to mimic the naturally occurring phenomenon with vaccines. Vaccines are killed or modified bad guys. Vaccines can't produce disease themselves, but they contain the offending antigen, the part that stimulates the body's immune system. As a result, vaccines cause the body to mount an immune response to the vaccine antigen and produce antibodies to it.

After an initial dose, most vaccines are followed by a booster dose. This makes sure that the body becomes well acquainted with the vaccine antigen and helps ensure that the highest possible antibody level is reached (taking advantage of the anamnestic response). Then, when an invader is encountered in real life and the horse's body is exposed to the natural antigen, the body has already been programmed to reach a high level of immunity against infection. This helps to fight off disease. Thus, vaccinations protect the body when confronted with a disease-producing agent.

VACCINATIONS: HOW OFTEN?

Two factors are very important in deciding how often you should vaccinate your horse. The first relates to how good an immune response is provoked by a vaccine. Some antigens, and therefore some vaccines, produce a stronger and more durable immune response than others. If a strong and long-lasting immune response is produced, you will not need to vaccinate the horse frequently to maintain a high level of antibodies in his blood. If the body's response to a vaccine is short term, however, more frequent vaccination will be needed to keep a high level of immunity.[2]

The other factor in deciding the frequency of vaccination for your horse is exposure. If you live in the middle of the desert and there are no other horses within a hundred miles and your horse never leaves the area, your horse is not likely to be exposed to very many disease-causing organisms. In this case, it's hard to defend mandating frequent vaccination against a variety of diseases, particularly contagious diseases that are spread by horse-to-horse contact. *Some* vaccinations will still be important, but this horse in the desert is not going to be exposed to many diseases.

On the other hand, if your horse lives in the middle of the city and he's in a facility where there are five hundred other horses and new horses are coming in and out of this place all the time, obviously the potential for exposure of your horse to new horses carrying different "germs" and to horses that may become sick is quite high. In this situation, it may be desirable to vaccinate your horse much more frequently and against more diseases than would be the case if he lived in the middle of the desert.

In this regard, horses are just like children. Any of you who have children know that sending them to school (where large groups of children tend to

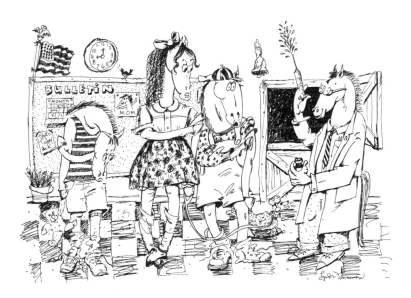

Regular vaccination is important for your horse.

gather reluctantly) is like issuing an invitation for the children to get sick. They promptly oblige and, in addition, bring the diseases home to share with the rest of the family. Thus, diseases spread.

A lot of the diseases that affect horses are like that, too. Get a bunch of horses together and there is a potential for them to develop and share diseases. Vaccinating your child is a good way to help prevent or lessen the severity of a number of illnesses. Vaccination does the same thing for your horse.

INFLUENZA

Influenza (flu) is a respiratory disease caused by a virus. The signs of influenza in horses are similar to those seen in people with a cold. The horse with influenza has a fever, cough and runny nose; won't eat; and generally feels lousy. He calls in sick and won't work. The disease is very contagious and spreads rapidly through a population of horses. Outbreaks involving 98 percent of horses in a facility, of all ages, have been reported.[3]

Influenza vaccine does not provoke a long-lasting immunity, only four to six months. After this time, there is no measurable level of protective antibodies in the blood. In light of this, it's kind of odd that most vaccine manufacturers recommend only annual boosters, after the initial two-shot series. It has been demonstrated that annual booster vaccination with the influenza vaccine does not provide protection against the influenza virus.[4,5,6,7]

Therefore, to make absolutely sure that your horse has a protective level of immunity against the influenza virus, you may have to vaccinate quite frequently, as much as every three or four months. Frequent vaccination is most important in horses at risk for exposure, such as horses going to shows, competitions or sales, or horses at breeding farms.[4] You may choose to vaccinate against influenza less often. Remember, the ideal vaccination schedule for your horse is influenced by many factors.

RHINOPNEUMONITIS

Rhinopneumonitis (another one of those medical school words—call it "rhino") is a name for another viral disease. Rhinopneumonitis is actually caused by *two* related viruses. They are members of a ubiquitous group of viruses known as herpes viruses. There are at least eight different strains of equine herpes virus that have been identified in horses, mules and donkeys.[8]

The two viruses that cause diseases in horses in the United States are responsible for the four different manifestations of this disease seen here. (There's another form seen elsewhere in the world.)

Form one causes respiratory disease. This form of rhino causes coldlike symptoms that clinically cannot be distinguished from influenza.

Form two affects the nervous system. You cannot protect against this form by vaccination. You can't cause it by vaccination, either. (Some people think that, but it's not true.) Fortunately, this form is quite rare. It is sometimes, but not always, fatal, and even severely affected horses that can't stand up have made full recoveries.[8]

Form three causes abortions late in pregnancy, during the last several months of gestation.

Form four causes foals that are near term to die in the uterus.

There are two types of vaccines against rhino.

For that matter, there are two types of vaccines against most anything. One type is a "killed" vaccine. This is, undoubtedly, the most commonly used type of vaccine against any disease. To make a killed vaccine, you take a virus, you kill it and then you vaccinate with it. Simple.

The other type of vaccine is a "modified live" vaccine. To make this type of vaccine, you take the virus and play with it. You take a horse respiratory virus, for instance, and grow it in rabbit spleen cells. The virus grows but becomes terribly confused (never having seen rabbit spleen cells, a most abnormal and upsetting situation for the virus). After a while in this unsettling environment, the virus loses its ability to produce disease in the horse, but it retains its ability to cause an antibody response. When the virus gets to this point, it can be made into a vaccine and reintroduced to the original host (the horse).[2]

The reason this is being brought up at all is that there are two types of rhino vaccines. One is generally thought to be best against the abortion form of the disease and the other is used more commonly to prevent the respiratory form. The killed virus is the only one recommended for helping to prevent abortion in pregnant mares, but it can also be used to help prevent the respiratory form of the disease. The modified live virus is recommended against respiratory disease but is not necessarily better at preventing it.[2]

Neither vaccine against rhino produces a long-lasting immunity—two to three months at the most. In pregnant mares, therefore, vaccination is recommended at five, seven and nine months of gestation, to provide protection against viral abortion late in the mare's term.

The fifth month of gestation, by the way, starts after 120 days of pregnancy. That's when mares should be vaccinated, not at 150 days, which is after the fifth month is over. Some people even advocate starting vaccination at three months.[9] It probably doesn't matter that much, as long as you follow a regular schedule. Unfortunately, abortion outbreaks have occurred even when all the mares have been regularly vaccinated.[8]

To protect against respiratory disease from the rhinopneumonitis virus and provide a measurable level of antibodies, vaccination needs to occur every two to three months. In this way, rhino is similar to flu.[8] These vaccines just do not provoke a long-lasting immunity.

There are combination products available with both flu and rhino in them. Consequently, the two vaccines are frequently given together in an effort to help stave off respiratory disease outbreaks.

TETANUS

Tetanus is caused by a toxin that is produced by bacteria. A toxin is a poison. In this case, the poison produced by the tetanus-causing bacteria is a protein that is very noxious. The bacteria live in the ground, and there's nothing that you can do about it. In wounds that are allowed to become infected, these bacteria can grow and die. As the bacteria die, their toxin is released into the system.

Tetanus is a particularly nasty disease in that the toxin affects the muscles and causes an untreatable but temporary spastic paralysis (you've undoubtedly heard it called lockjaw. That's because the muscles of the jaw become locked shut from the violent muscle contractions).

Tetanus is *not* always fatal, however.

Anyway, the immunity level produced by the tetanus vaccine is extremely strong and long lasting. The protection from a single vaccine may last five to ten years, similar to the situation in people.[10] But because horses live in dirt and shavings and manure, almost everyone recommends a yearly booster.[11]

The tetanus myth is that horses get tetanus at the drop of a hat and you have to vaccinate them against tetanus whenever they scrape themselves or sometimes even if your clippers get a little too close. No. A once-a-year tetanus vaccination is more than enough to provide good protection against this disease.

TETANUS TOXOID VS. TETANUS ANTITOXIN

There is considerable confusion about the two tetanus products available for horses, tetanus toxoid and antitoxin. The toxoid is what is used annually to vaccinate horses to prevent the disease. Much like the virus that has been changed by growing it in abnormal host cells, a toxoid is a "changed" toxin. The toxoid vaccine retains its ability to provoke an immune response but loses its ability to produce disease.

On the other hand, when a horse is given tetanus antitoxin, it is just like giving him an instant dose of antibodies. If blood serum (the liquid part, without the cells) is obtained from a horse that has been made resistant to tetanus by vaccination and if this serum is given to a second horse with no previous history of vaccination or exposure, then the second horse will also become temporarily resistant to tetanus (until the administered serum grows old). The serum from the vaccinated horse provides some antibodies to help prevent disease in the unvaccinated horse. Tetanus antitoxin does the same thing.[2]

Antitoxin treatment might occasionally be important to give to a wounded horse that has never been exposed to a tetanus vaccine, to provide some immediate protection from the tetanus toxin, or in a baby that didn't get immune factors from his mother's milk.[11] More on that in a minute. In a horse that has been vaccinated, however, the body produces its anamnestic response so quickly and to such a high level that giving antitoxin isn't necessary.

Not only that, but giving a horse tetanus antitoxin can occasionally be dangerous. If antitoxin is given to a horse with an already high immune level, an immune reaction known as serum sickness can occur. When this happens, the unfortunate result can be kidney failure.[2] That's not to say that antitoxin will kill your horse, but the safest thing to do is to start with the tetanus toxoid and stick with it. It will provide your horse with good protection.

Horse owners seem frantic to protect their horses from tetanus, especially new babies. Consequently, many baby horses are given a "tetanus shot" within hours of being born. This isn't needed.

That's right, you don't need to give a shot of the toxoid (or the antitoxin) to your newborn foal. Why? Because they can't respond to the toxoid and the antitoxin is unnecessary. The foal gets high levels of antibodies to tetanus (and many other illnesses) from the mare's first milk (known as the colostrum). These high levels *prevent* the foal from being able to respond to the tetanus toxoid vaccine. The vaccine has no effect in these young foals. Furthermore, since the colostrum provides circulating antibodies for the foal, there's no need for the antitoxin, either.[13] Plus, the antitoxin can give the foal serum sickness.

The best way to protect your newborn foal against tetanus is to vaccinate the mare with tetanus toxoid one month before she foals. This will cause an anamnestic (see how these words come back to haunt you?) response to tetanus in the mare. As a result, she will increase the level of tetanus antibodies in her milk. The foal will then receive protection against tetanus when he nurses. You can start vaccinating your baby at two to three months of age, when the immunity from the milk starts to wear off and the foal is able to respond to the stimulus of the tetanus vaccine (as well as the others that are given).

Therefore, in neonates, in the single instance where the foal did not obtain adequate immune factors from the mare's milk (there are tests for this) or if the mare has never been vaccinated against tetanus (which, given the fact that horses can't seem to get through a week without getting a tetanus shot, is unlikely), administration of tetanus antitoxin may be advisable.[13] But that's it.

One other thing. Although vaccination against tetanus is extremely important in horses, the bacteria can't live in normal, healthy tissue.[12] If your horse sustains some sort of a wound, take care of it. If you make sure your horse's wound doesn't get infected, he won't develop tetanus.

ENCEPHALITIS

Encephalitis (sleeping sickness) is a viral disease of the nervous system. Nervous system diseases have really weird signs, and they vary among horses. Some sick horses show extreme depression, compulsive walking and head pressing. Others can be excitable or aggressive. These diseases are, unfortunately, often (but not always) fatal.

There are several strains of encephalitis virus. The strains that occur in the United States are called Eastern and Western. There is also a Venezuelan strain that lives in Mexico and south of Mexico and has, once, about twenty years ago, crossed into Texas (where it was promptly lassoed and eradicated). Venezuelan encephalitis doesn't occur in the United States.

The encephalitis vaccine gives an immunity that lasts for six to eight months.[14] Sleeping sickness virus is carried by biting insects, most commonly mosquitos, so you need to make sure that when you vaccinate against encephalitis, adequate levels of immunity are present to cover the mosquito season. Vaccinating against encephalitis in October in Minnesota isn't particularly useful.

Vaccinating against *Venezuelan* encephalitis is not necessarily a good idea, however. First of all, since the disease hasn't been seen in the United States for twenty years, there's no good reason to protect against it. Second, and perhaps more important, if your horse has a titer (blood level) against Venezuelan encephalitis, you may not be able to export him to certain other countries where the disease does not occur. It doesn't matter to the importing country if your horse got his titer from being vaccinated. For all they know, he was exposed to Venezuelan encephalitis. It's impossible to tell if a titer comes from vaccination or exposure to disease. A country that doesn't have Venezuelan encephalitis doesn't want it. If there is any indication that your horse was exposed to this disease, another country may not let him in. Since most horses don't travel to foreign countries, this probably won't be a big deal, but if you are involved in international competition, this caveat is an important thing to remember.

At this point, it might be useful to sum up the information you have so far. Tetanus and encephalitis don't require other horses to be around for your horse to get them. What does this mean? You should vaccinate once a year with a product containing the vaccine against Eastern and Western encephalitis (to cover the mosquito season) and that also prevents tetanus to make sure that your horse doesn't get that disease, either.

In situations where many horses are kept close together, it may be appropriate to vaccinate much more frequently, perhaps as often as every two or three months, to protect your horse against the viral diseases of influenza and rhinopneumonitis. These respiratory diseases are spread by direct contact with other horses and can also move a short distance through the air.

Have you ever noticed how people love to give catchy names to things? New York City is the "Big Apple." Optical art becomes "op art." That sort of thing. When you combine flu, tetanus and Eastern and Western encephalitis you get a "four-way" vaccine. (In cattle, there are "seven-way" vaccines, the components of which need not be listed here.) "Four-way" products are very common. If you add something else to the "four-way" mix, you have a "five-way" vaccine. Whatever.

POTOMAC HORSE FEVER

Potomac horse fever first reared its head in the early 1980s, in the Potomac River area of Maryland and Virginia. The term was coined by a television reporter, and now it's part of the same horse lore that gave us terms like "windpuffs." Anyway, this is a nasty disease that can cause fever, depression, loss of appetite, diarrhea, laminitis and, if untreated (and sometimes when treated), death. Any one of these signs may be seen in a sick horse, but rarely does one horse show them all. Recently, a second form of this disease, which causes mares to abort, has also been recognized.[15]

The initial vaccine is followed by a booster dose three or four weeks later. A yearly booster is recommended by the manufacturer, but as with the influenza virus, that may not be enough to protect your horse. In fact, field observations suggest that only about 50 percent of vaccinated horses may be protected six months after vaccination.[16] To provide an adequate protective level of immunity, some authorities recommend that you vaccinate every four months.[15] The vaccine has been reported to be about 78 percent effective in preventing the disease in experimental situations[17] and it *has* reduced the overall occurrence of the disease in horses. All of the above applies to the form of Potomac horse fever that causes horses to get sick; the effect of vaccination on preventing abortion in mares isn't known. Even after much research, the disease is a bit of a mystery—no one knows how it is spread—but fortunately the vaccine has been helpful in reducing and controlling its occurrence.

RABIES

Some horses are vaccinated against rabies, especially east of the Rocky Mountains. Rabies is invariably fatal and causes some really weird nervous system signs in horses. Unlike the classic symptoms in dogs, horses do not generally become aggressive, biting beasts when they contract rabies (although there is a "furious" form). Rather, they tend to become very depressed and/or uncoordinated.[18] Unfortunately, the signs of rabies can be mixed up with other diseases of the nervous system, and the likelihood of making an accurate diagnosis before the horse dies is pretty much impossible. There are no blood or blood chemistry tests to help make a diagnosis.

In areas of the country where rabies occurs, rabies vaccination is very important for your horse. Although vaccination is a very effective way to prevent the disease, vaccine breaks have occurred.[18] After initial vaccinations, a yearly booster is recommended.

BOTULISM

In central Kentucky horses are commonly vaccinated against botulism (the disease can occur in other places but outbreaks elsewhere have been very rare). Botulism, like tetanus, is caused by a bacterial toxin, but it causes death by a flaccid muscle paralysis (just the opposite of tetanus). A horse that gets botulism and isn't treated will almost always die. Botulism is a type of food poisoning, that is, foals and horses can pick the toxin up from stagnant water or from contaminated feed.

Fortunately, the vaccine has proven fairly effective in preventing the disease. It is given three times, two weeks to four weeks apart (depending on who's doing it). Giving the vaccine to mares in foal will help prevent botulism (shaker foal syndrome) in the new babies once they're born. A yearly booster is required to keep up the immunity.

As with tetanus, there's a botulism antitoxin, too. It is given to horses when they are sick with botulism, and if given early enough, it's pretty effective at helping save them.[19] Talk about expensive, though: Treatment with botulism antitoxin costs thousands of dollars. Conversely, how much would it be worth to you to save your horse's life?

ENDOTOXIN

Endotoxins are released from certain types of bacteria when they die. They can cause horses to get very sick when given experimentally, but their role in naturally occurring disease isn't clear. There is a vaccine available for use against them but its efficacy has yet to be determined.

EQUINE VIRAL ARTERITIS

Equine viral arteritis is a disease that has been around a long time but has recently gotten a lot of press. Like influenza and rhinopneumonitis, it's a viral disease that can spread rapidly through groups of horses. Horses sick with this disease show fever, depression and limb stiffness, among other signs. The thing that usually alerts people to viral arteritis is the fact that sick horses tend to swell up. Swelling can occur in the legs, face, shoulder, belly or pretty much anywhere. Abortions in mares can occur, too.

Most people think that this is a really bad disease. It isn't. In fact, death from naturally occurring cases of equine viral arteritis is pretty rare, even when the horses aren't treated.[20]

The biggest problem with viral arteritis is that it can cause stallions to become carriers of the disease, possibly even for the lifetime of the stallion.[21] Accordingly, stallions that are exported to certain countries have to be tested. Many stallions in affected areas are carriers of the disease and they can't be exported. This has cost some stallion owners millions of dollars.[22]

There's a good vaccine available against viral arteritis. It provides strong clinical protection against the disease, at least one to three years.[20] The vaccine presents one big problem, though. If you vaccinate your horse against viral arteritis, you risk him always having a blood level of antibodies against the disease. Much as with Venezuelan encephalitis, if your horse has a titer against equine viral arteritis, you may not be able to ship him to other countries that don't have the disease because they will not be able to tell if he got his titer from vaccination or from contracting the disease. Ask your veterinarian if you are concerned that you need to vaccinate against this disease.

STRANGLES

Strangles is another disease you've undoubtedly heard of. The vaccine against it, however, doesn't work very well. This disease is so misunderstood and has generated so many myths that it is the subject of an entire chapter (see Chapter 11).

VACCINE REACTIONS

Unfortunately, horses sometimes have reactions to vaccines. Vaccines can make horses feel sick. They can cause local swelling and pain at the injection site, and in severe cases they can cause local abscesses. Most of the time this is an unavoidable and unforeseen response from a particular horse rather than a problem with the vaccine. Many vaccine reactions may be caused by an adjuvant that may have been added to the vaccine.

An adjuvant is a substance that enhances the immune response. Experimentally it has been demonstrated that adding certain substances to a vaccine can make the immune response stronger, although veterinarians don't really know why it does.[2] Sometimes these substances can provoke a local tissue reaction in the horse. Vaccine reactions usually pass fairly quickly, and although they are irritating to you and the horse, they are generally not a health threat.

Some people think that you have to give the horse a day off after vaccination. There is no medical reason for this. In fact, a good case can be made for vigorous exercise right after vaccination. Exercise increases the heart rate, which will increase the circulatory rate, which should speed the removal of the vaccine from the site where it was deposited in the muscle. This could conceivably help decrease the incidence of vaccine reaction.

So why the day off? The author has observed that when horses do have a reaction to a vaccine, the owner of the horse frequently panics. He or she will call, sometimes at odd hours of the night, to discuss the situation. The author believes that if the owner is advised not to ride the horse the next day, there is a decreased likelihood that the horse will be seen by the owner on that day. If the horse has a reaction, therefore, he will not be seen by the owner, who will, happily, not get worried. If the owner isn't worried, the veterinarian will not get a frantic call, interrupting an otherwise busy working day. As an added benefit, resting horses on the day after vaccination allows horse trainers to enjoy a day off to go play golf (or something else) following vaccination of all the horses in the barn.

The "right" vaccination program for your horse is influenced by the area in which you live and your horse's potential for exposure to disease-causing organisms. Your veterinarian should be a good source of information about which diseases are prevalent in your area and which should therefore be protected against by vaccination.

Remember that vaccinations are not a foolproof way to keep your horse from ever getting sick. The invaders that cause disease have the ability to modify their structures. New strains can perfectly well sidestep the immunity obtained by vaccination. Also, sometimes horses get sick in spite of good vaccine programs.

Vaccination can never be a substitute for the important measures of isolation of infected animals and good, clean hygienic conditions and methods of operation. If you have a large stable, for instance, while it is a good idea to require vaccinations prior to allowing a horse to enter your facility, it is also a good idea to quarantine him for a month or so to help keep him from spreading any disease that he might be developing. If a sick horse has been in a stall, the stall should be cleaned thoroughly with disinfectants prior to putting a new horse in the stall. Don't trust vaccines to do all the work of preventing diseases.

There are some general rules that you *can* follow. Vaccinate your horse at least once a year with a tetanus and encephalitis product. Protect him frequently against flu and rhino if he lives in crowded conditions. Protect him against rabies, botulism, viral arteritis and Potomac horse fever if these diseases occur in your area. Ask your veterinarian about endotoxins. Read the chapter about strangles and then decide for yourself what to do about this disease. Vaccinations can't prevent all the problems that horses have, but they can go a long way toward helping horses stay healthy.

8

Deworming

As part of preventive maintenance for horses, people also deworm them. Please note: People deworm horses. They do not give them worms—that is, "worm" them. (This is just a pet peeve.) Horses, it seems, are the host for a variety of internal parasites. The majority of these parasites ("worms") lay eggs inside the horse and then get passed out in the manure. They lie in egg stage on the ground until they are picked up by another horse, either from blades of grass that are contaminated or from just eating manure (which horses enjoy doing, as you have recently learned). The eggs then mature inside the nice, warm horse and ultimately the adult worms begin to lay eggs, which starts the cycle all over again.

Not all horse parasites follow this pattern of growth. Some parasites haven't read the book on this type of life cycle and choose to follow another. This is very interesting to parasitologists. It is not very interesting to anyone else.

People are either "splitters" or "lumpers." There are twenty or so internal parasites of the horse. The "splitters" want to know about each and every internal parasite. The "lumpers" are content to realize that horses get worms and that deworming products kill them. The author is a lumper. For you splitters, there are a variety of texts on the subject.[1]

PARASITES AND THEIR EFFECTS

Internal parasites are associated with a number of problems in the horse. First, they can cause horses to look unhealthy and unthrifty. The worms get some of the nutrition that was rightfully meant for the horse. It takes quite a load of parasites to cause weight loss in a horse, however.

Second, parasites have been associated with colics. One type of parasite, *Strongylus vulgaris*, undergoes one of its developmental stages in one of the major arteries that supplies the large intestines. It is thought that these larvae can clog circulation to the intestine and are therefore thought to be associated with a type of colic known as thromboembolic colic. In this type of colic, the larvae present in the arteries cause blood clots to form, presumably because they interfere with the blood flow. The blood clots (thrombi) can then break off and travel down the affected artery (the traveling clots are called emboli). The emboli then plug up the local circulation and cause the intestine to become unhealthy in the area that has its blood supply reduced or cut off.[2] Another parasite, the tapeworm, has been associated with a different type of colic in the horse, one in which segments of bowel slip up into each other like the parts of a telescope. This is called an intussusception (a magnificent medical word).[3]

Third, one of the parasites that didn't read the book about how parasite life cycles are supposed to go (causing extra work for veterinary students everywhere), *Onchocerca,* has a stage that lives in the horse's skin. Roughly 10 percent of horses can develop an allergic reaction to this parasite, which causes the skin to get crusty in a few characteristic areas (like the neck, ears and midline of the belly) and makes horses itch like crazy.

Finally, another parasite, *Habronema*, will sometimes get confused. This one has yet another life cycle. *Habronema* eggs are supposed to be laid in the mucous membranes of the mouth. Problems can happen, however, when instead of laying its eggs in the mucous membranes of the mouth like it is supposed to, the parasite deposits the eggs in the mucous membranes of the eye or the penis. When this happens, the eggs can't develop normally and the result is a granuloma (a dollar word for a big red mass of inflamed tissue).

Parasites certainly can cause problems for horses, but what is more certain is that they give horse owners fits. The "best" way to kill these creatures is subject for countless research papers and presumably endless hours of stall-side discussion, but any number of ways are pretty effective. (You knew that there was not going to be a straight answer, didn't you?)

DEWORMING COMPOUNDS

First, a word about the deworming compounds themselves. A big myth says that deworming compounds are dangerous chemicals and that the slightest overdose can send a horse into a toxic reaction from which he may never recover. This may have been true back when horses were dewormed with things like tobacco and whiskey. Whiskey and tobacco can be very dangerous when given to horses. (They are very dangerous when given to people, too, but that has not deterred their use.) Modern deworming compounds are not at all dangerous.

Most deworming compounds work because the metabolism of a worm is very different from that of a horse. All living things function using chemical reactions. The chemicals that make the worm function do not exist in the horse. Therefore, scientists have been able to design chemicals that are specifically targeted at the worm's system. These chemicals are extremely toxic to the worm but have virtually no effect on the horse because there's nothing in the horse that the chemicals affect. Most deworming products are safe at a dose of forty times more than the horse is supposed to get. This is almost impossible to do, unless you have a lot of time on your hands and unlimited funds. The point is, these products are really safe.[4]

Except for one (of course). There are deworming products on the market that have in them a type of chemical called an organophosphate. The products that contain it generally advertise that they *specifically* kill parasites known as bots. Read the label on the product to see if it has dichlorvos or trichlorfon in it. These compounds are generally safe if dosed at the manufacturer's recommended level; however, adverse reactions *can* occur at the recommended dose.[4] These are older types of deworming products, and there's really no reason to use them at all. Products that contain ivermectin control bots and other parasites with a much wider margin of safety. If you do use organophosphates, watch the dose.

Ivermectin has taken the parasite control world by storm since its introduction in the early 1980s. It kills all worms except tapeworms, and it even kills the baby worms (larvae) before they grow into adults. It even kills the worms that live normally in the skin (*Onchocerca*) and abnormally in the mucous membranes (*Habronema*).

Benzimidazoles (oxibendazole, fenbendazole, mebendazole and the like) have been around for a long time. They do a good job on most of the worms but don't kill tapeworms or the ones in the stomach (bots) and mucous membranes. Given at a high dose, or on successive days, some members of this class can kill the baby worms, too. Some parasites show resistance to some members of this class of dewormers, but parasite resistance is not a major problem. These drugs are very safe and generally effective. A related chemical class of deworming products is known as febantel. This product is metabolized by the horse's body to become a benzimidazole and it works the same way as these drugs, with the same pluses and minuses.

Pyrantel pamoate is a good drug, too. It is the only one that kills tapeworms, but you have to double the recommended dose to do it (give the horse two tubes of medication). It doesn't kill the worms in the skin nor does it get the bots. Parasite resistance has not been a significant problem with these drugs.

Piperazine is an older deworming product that is used by some practitioners, primarily against ascarids, parasites affecting younger horses. It is safe and works well, but other products have a much broader range of activity and thus are more commonly used.

A final class, levamisole, is not widely used because it is relatively toxic and not particularly effective against some of the more prevalent equine parasites. It's listed here for completeness; don't ask your veterinarian to deworm your horse with levamisole, or he or she will look at you funny.

DEWORMING METHODS

The biggest problem with establishing a deworming program for most people is that they have so many choices. Wouldn't it be nice if you could just get a straight, easy answer to a question like "What's the best program?" As long as you use something that's effective and use it periodically, you're going to kill a lot of worms. Clearly, though, this will not help you talk about worms stall-side and handle all of the myths and misconceptions.

Here's one of the biggest myths about deworming: "The route of administration matters." Or to put it another way, "You have to have your horse dewormed by a nasogastric tube (tube wormed) every once in a while."

Well, that's just ridiculous.

Back before the existence of effective paste and feed dewormers, some rationale existed for shoving a tube up your horse's nose in order to administer deworming medication to him. That is no longer the case.

You can give deworming medication to your horse in three ways. Some dewormers can be mixed with your horse's feed (one brand of these you give every day and yes, it's very safe). You can give your horse a deworming paste in his mouth. Or you can pass a tube up his nose and down his esophagus and deposit a liquid dewormer in the vicinity of his stomach. (There was an injectable deworming product, but it was pulled from the market in 1984.)

This is important. *All methods of administration are equally effective, assuming two things:* First, the horse must get the proper dose for his weight. Deworming a twelve-hundred-pound horse with a thousand-pound dose of dewormer doesn't work efficiently, whatever the method of administration. If you have any question about your horse's weight, overdose him. The products are safe, and what are you going to do with a teeny little bit of leftover dewormer, anyway? Second, and this is really obvious, for the deworming product to be effective the horse must get the whole dose. If you take a tube of deworming paste and squirt it at the horse and half of it ends up on your spouse or significant other, the product is not going to work. But if you get those two little things done, then there is no difference in effectiveness between any of the deworming products. Study after study has demonstrated this.[1,4,5,6]

Why does this myth about deworming by nasogastric tube persist? Is it because people believe that veterinarians have "stronger" dewormers than the ones that they can buy? (They don't.) Is it because people believe it's important to deliver the medication "right to the site"? (It isn't important and tube deworming doesn't do that anyway. The tube gets down close to the stomach and the worms are as much as eighty feet or so down the gut.) Is it because people don't want to change the way that they've done things for a hundred years? (You're getting warmer.) Is it because people don't read the current research? (Hope not.)

You may feel it's necessary to run a tube up your horse's nose periodically for some reason. The horse wouldn't agree, and neither do the researchers. There's no *medical* reason to do it.

THE DEWORMING SCHEDULE

Well, if the method of deworming isn't important, how about the schedule of dewormers? Should they be rotated or should one product be given for a year, then switched? Or does it matter?

It probably doesn't matter that much. There is no firm evidence that rotating deworming products either prevents or promotes resistance to these drugs. No deworming product or deworming schedule is 100 percent effective in killing and controlling all the worms of the horse, and occasional resistance to some dewormers has been found in some worms. It does make sense that prolonged use of one single product would tend to select for a strain of parasite resistant to that one product. Since no dewormer kills all the worms, it makes sense that you should use each of them occasionally.

HOW OFTEN?

The majority of the worms of adult horses have a life cycle of six to eleven months, which is the time it takes for the worms to reach maturity after they are ingested. To control them, you need to kill worms regularly and to interrupt their life cycle so that your horse won't keep scattering eggs all over the place.

In adult horses, the frequency of deworming is primarily determined by exposure. Lush, moist pastures are ideal conditions for parasite eggs to survive. Parasite eggs can cause reinfestation in the horse for up to a year. If lots of horses live together in these conditions, there is a terrific opportunity for parasites to spread among them. If your horse is exposed to lots of parasites, you need to deworm often—even as often as every four to six weeks—because new adults are going to be entering your horse's intestines all the time. If you really want to deworm your horse often, one of the feed dewormers is given daily.[5]

If, however, your horse lives in a desert or is kept in a stall and can't get to other horses' manure, the potential for him to pick up internal parasites is pretty slight. Your horse can be dewormed every three or four months and will probably be just fine.

The newest approach to deworming is to try to control them seasonally. With this method, deworming is scheduled to try to kill the egg-laying adults when they are at their highest numbers inside the horse. In the northern two-thirds of the United States, there is typically a rise in numbers of strongyle-type parasites in the spring. By deworming horses in the spring and early summer, parasite transmission is reduced because the adults are killed before they can lay eggs. This technique only works where this seasonal rise in parasites is known to occur, however.[5] Ask your veterinarian for advice on establishing a deworming schedule.

In *young* horses, up to two years of age, it is especially important to control ascarids. As opposed to the parasites of adult horses, the ascarid develops fairly rapidly, taking about sixty days for the life cycle to complete itself from egg to egg-laying adult. The immature forms of this parasite migrate through the liver and lungs of the young horse and damage them, especially the lungs. Ascarid larvae are associated with the development of pneumonia in these little guys.[7] Ascarid control is fairly important in foals. It is generally recommended that young horses be dewormed every sixty days, starting at two months of age, with a product that kills ascarids (most do). Apparently, as horses get older they develop some immunity to ascarids and so, after the horse passes his second year, it's not as important to target these worms specifically.[8]

OTHER METHODS OF CONTROL

Deworming is not the only effective way to help control parasites. In fact, it may not even be the best way. In addition to chemical deworming, other methods of parasite control should be used when possible. Measures can be taken to help control the transmission of the parasite eggs, for example. Simple measures such as plowing or reseeding fields can be very hard on parasite populations. Making grass into hay is very destructive to parasite larvae, and spreading of manure can leave larvae unprotected against hostile environments. In hot, dry climates, the eggs that are thus exposed to the environment dry out and die rapidly. But manure spreading can be something of a double-edged sword. In lush, moist conditions manure spreading can distribute parasite eggs all over the place, so be careful.

Removal of manure from pasture is a great way to keep horses from being parasitized. Studies have shown that this actually works better at controlling parasites than does chemical deworming.[9,10] Pastures can literally be vacuumed of manure, using mechanical vacuums, or the manure can be picked up with a rake. Some people have even advocated the use of sheep and cattle as "biological" vacuum cleaners. Allowed to graze on horse pasture, sheep and cattle will happily eat up horse parasite eggs along with the grass. This poses no threat to sheep and cows, since horse parasites cannot infect them, but the effectiveness of this method of parasite control is questionable.[10] Sheep and cattle do give a wonderful down home feeling to your pasture or paddock, however.

MONITORING THE PROGRAM

To monitor the effectiveness of your deworming program, you can have your horse's manure checked for parasite eggs. This is a reasonably effective way to see how your deworming program is going, but unfortunately many internal parasites do not shed eggs regularly. A single manure sample may not be an accurate reflection of your horse's parasite level. You'll need several consecutive manure samples to obtain meaningful results from analysis of the manure.[11]

BOTS

A brief word about bots. Bots are parasites that live in the horse's stomach. In the parts of the country where they occur (almost everywhere except a desert), the adult botfly buzzes around the horse's legs and makes the horse nuts. The fly looks something like a big bee. The botfly lays its eggs on the horse's legs. Botfly eggs are bright yellow, and if your horse is being bothered by them, you will see all sorts of little yellow specks in the hair of your horse's legs. The horse licks the eggs off in the course of normal horse activity, which thus perpetuates the life cycle of the parasite. The ingested larvae attach in the horse's stomach and are quite happy there.

Bots apparently don't cause much damage to the horse, but people hate them and want to get rid of them. Generally, it is recommended to wait until about thirty days after the first killing frost to deworm for bots, although some people recommend more frequent deworming. Thirty days after the first killing frost, horses won't get reinfested with bots because the adult flies are all dead (they have no tolerance for cold weather). So if you only deworm for bots once, do it then. If you use ivermectin a lot as part of your regular deworming program, you'll be killing lots of bots all the time, so you probably don't have to worry about it much.[12]

Use deworming products regularly, as your horse's exposure level dictates. Change the products every once in a while. Make sure the horse gets all of his deworming medicine. Give him the proper dose for his weight and overdose him if you're not sure. In addition to chemical deworming compounds, use other methods to control parasites, where appropriate. If you do all of this, everything will undoubtedly be just fine.

9

Teeth

Another thing veterinarians regularly look at (and owners regularly worry about) is the horse's teeth. Horse teeth change with time. Not fast, mind you, but they do erupt steadily over the course of the horse's life. Horse teeth also overlap each other on the sides. Viewed from the front of the mouth to the back, the upper teeth hang out over the outside edge of the lower teeth, and the lower teeth overlap the inside edge of the upper teeth. This means the outside edge of the upper teeth and the inside edge of the lower teeth don't have opposing surfaces.

As the horse chews, the teeth grind down against each other. This grinding of the teeth is part of normal tooth wear and keeps the exposed teeth at a relatively constant length during the horse's life. Since the edges that overlap on the upper and lower teeth don't have a surface to rest against or grind against, however, these edges tend not to wear down as much as the rest of the tooth. Over time, this can lead to the formation of sharp edges, or "points," on the sides of the horse's teeth.

Because points form, people want to file the teeth down so that the edges are smooth. This is called "floating" the teeth, although it's not at all clear why it's called that. The points that form on horse teeth are a subject for some discussion around the barns because people worry that their horses won't be able to eat if they have points on their teeth. This may eventually happen in the wild. If a horse lives twenty-five years in the wild and manages to avoid coyotes and gopher holes, his teeth may become quite sharp and long. As such, they may eventually cause him some discomfort when he eats because his now abnormal teeth might interfere with his ability to chew. It appears that they rarely do, but they *might*. Reports of domesticated horses losing weight because of abnormal teeth have been few, probably because people pay so much attention to them. (In elephants, by the way, the wearing out of the teeth is thought to be a contributing factor to the death of older elephants. So far, no one has been bold enough to float an elephant's teeth.)

If you get your horse's teeth checked once a year or so and have the points filed down when they get sharp, your horse will most likely never have a problem with his teeth. Horse teeth erupt very slowly (approximately 2.2 millimeters per year) and once a year is more than enough to have them checked. This is true even if your horse's teeth are put into his head in an irregular fashion, such as occurs with "wavemouthed" horses.[1]

Viewed from the side, teeth can overlap from front to back, too. Much as the sides that overlap can develop sharp points, the areas that don't match up from front to back can grow up or down (depending on which tooth doesn't match up) and cause hooks on the teeth. Regular tooth floating can control the growth of these hooks, but if they go unrecognized they may have to be cut off. It takes the better part of a day to file down since they're so hard. The device to do this, called a molar cutter, looks something like a bolt cutter and is really quite cumbersome and impressive. Watching someone try to use a molar cutter can be a lively source of entertainment for everyone around except for the horse and the operator of the equipment. If hooks go unrecognized they can eventually give the horse problems in closing his mouth or chewing, but neither will happen very quickly or at an early age. The easiest way to tell if your horse has hooks is to look in his mouth. If you don't want to look in your horse's mouth, you can get a good idea if he has hooks or is going to develop them by looking at how the front teeth, the incisors, line up. A horse with a prominent overbite ("parrot mouth") or underbite ("monkey mouth") will tend to have back teeth (molars and premolars) that don't match up either (but not always). These are the teeth that eventually get hooks.[1]

TEETH FLOATING

Because teeth change so slowly, teeth floating is never an emergency. And teeth should never have to be floated very often, either.

You could get into arguments about the right way to float a horse's teeth. Teeth floating is not especially difficult nor is it a great test of one's veterinary ability. That being said, all sorts of people (veterinarians and otherwise) assert that they can and should float a horse's teeth and that theirs is the "best" or "only" way to do so. There is no "best" way to float a horse's teeth any more than there is a "best" way to wash your car, but using a device to hold the horse's mouth open can help make sure that even those teeth in the back of the mouth get smoothed down. Any veterinarian who is conscientious should be able to do a good job of smoothing and leveling the horse's teeth.

Since you are unlikely to stick your hand into your horse's mouth to feel the teeth for yourself (although it's not hard), you are most likely going to rely on the good graces of someone else to tell when it's necessary to have your horse's teeth floated. This puts you in a precarious position, since you are at the mercy of whoever is checking your horse's teeth to tell you if they need to be floated. Pick someone who's honest and reliable to look in your horse's mouth and not someone who's out to take advantage of a relatively easy opportunity to make some money. Get your horse's teeth checked every once in a while, and if you remember that floating shouldn't need to be done very often you'll protect yourself from overeager tooth floaters.

BAD TEETH AND WEIGHT LOSS

People think that bad teeth are the primary cause of weight loss in the horse. This just isn't so. The number one cause of weight loss in horses is that they don't get enough to eat. Bad teeth *have* been associated with weight loss in the horse, but if your horse has had semiregular dental care and is losing weight, the problem is almost undoubtedly somewhere else.

BABY TEETH

Young horses lose teeth (just like young anything else), and way too much attention is paid to this. Most horses will lose their baby teeth without help from horse owners, but being people and wanting to help, owners invariably worry about such things. In the normal situation, the permanent teeth grow up from under the baby teeth and push them right on out the mouth. The baby teeth in the front (the incisors) shed from the center out, at approximately two and a half, three and a half and four and a half years of age, respectively. Therefore, not only should you not be alarmed when these teeth start falling out, you should also have a pretty good idea of how old your horse is. It is possible for the baby teeth to be retained in the horse, and they are very easily removed.[2,3]

The first cheek teeth (premolars) also shed, but they grow out a bit differently. These teeth are tightly packed together, and you'll never notice that anything is loose back there. You'll most likely never know when or if the baby

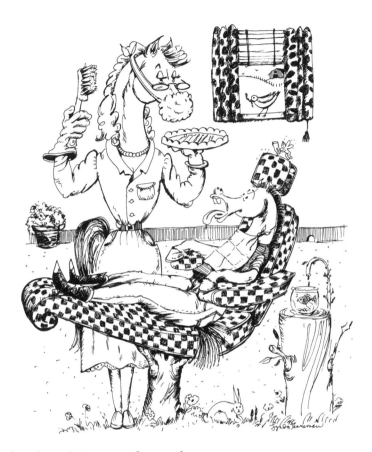

Regular dental care is important for your horse.

premolars are coming out. The permanent teeth start growing in from behind these baby teeth at about two and a half years, and they snuggle right up against the baby tooth (which fits perfectly on top of the permanent tooth) and push it on out. If the baby tooth doesn't drop right out and hangs on, it is referred to as a cap.[1] This can be knocked out with a screwdriver or something if you want, but most of the time the caps just fall off and you never see them, unless they show up in the feed bin.

TEETH AND THE BRIDLE

Teeth *can* evidently cause some problems with a horse's bridle. When you tighten the bridle onto his cheeks some discomfort can occur if the inside of the cheeks rub against sharp teeth. Check for sharp points if your horse starts tossing his head for no reason and get the points filed down if they exist.

Many times, however, you can't tell if your horse resents his bridle because he needs his teeth floated until after the fact. You could probably solicit a number of opinions as to whether the teeth *are* too sharp or not, but the only real way that you're ever going to know if they *were* too sharp is to file them down and see if there's any difference in your horse's behavior. Then you'll know if the teeth were a problem (and if they weren't, at least you won't have to worry about the teeth for a while).

WOLF TEETH

Wolf teeth are little bitty teeth, right at the front of the big cheek teeth, which occur in some (but not all) horses. These are not the canine teeth, which sit by themselves on the sides of most horse's mouths, behind the front teeth and in front of the big cheek teeth. Canine teeth really don't cause any problems, although sometimes people will tell you that they are too sharp. You can file them down or cut them off if you are so inclined. Sometimes people want to have the canines removed, thinking that they are wolf teeth. The roots on these things go down to the hooves. Extraction is no easy feat and is almost never necessary.[2]

The wolf teeth most likely don't cause any problems for the horse, either, but a lot of trainers like to have them removed because they are convinced that they cause horses problems with the bit. Trainers swear that the bit hits the horse in the wolf teeth, causing irritation. Due to the location of the wolf teeth, the fact that they have almost nonexistent roots to get irritated and the fact that a properly fitting bridle should not get anywhere near them, it seems unlikely that the presence of wolf teeth is a real problem.[1] It might be best to go along with this anachronism when your trainer insists on pulling them, however, just so that you don't get him or her mad at you. Sometimes it's just not worth bucking the system. Many horses have wolf teeth and have no problems with them at all.

TEETH AND AGE

It has been fairly commonly accepted that a trained observer can accurately age the horse by looking at his incisor teeth and noting characteristic changes that correlate to each year of age. There are even books and charts on this subject. However, a recent study in England that compared the actual known ages of over 400 horses to their ages estimated by looking at the teeth showed that veterinarians were unable to age horses by their teeth with any accuracy at all after five years of age![4] A set of registration papers, when available, is a much more accurate source of information about your horse's age than his teeth.

EQUINE "DENTISTS"

The best source of information about your horse's teeth is your veterinarian. He or she is the only one out there who has medical training in horse health. Other people may represent themselves as teeth "specialists," but there are no training programs for equine "dentists" that are even remotely comparable to the training required for human dentistry. These programs at best involve a few days of training, as opposed to the many years of schooling that are required for a human dentist. Just as there are untrained horse "chiropractors" who take advantage of the name of chiropractic, many equine "dentists" are just people who (we hope) have learned how to float teeth and pull wolf teeth. In the author's experience, many of these technicians can do only that because these particular things are not especially difficult to learn or do. These people may not be trained to recognize more significant problems.

In many states, someone who works independently as an equine "dentist" is actually breaking the law. The care of horse teeth is part of the practice of veterinary medicine. Examination and treatment of the horse's mouth by untrained and unlicensed people is considered, in most states, the practicing of veterinary medicine without a license and it is illegal. In these states, however, a dental technician *can* work in conjunction with and under the supervision of a veterinarian, just as an animal health technician in a small-animal veterinarian's office can draw blood from your dog. Beware, though, of "dentists" who tell you that all horses need to have their teeth floated several times a year or that veterinarians don't know how to do the job. That's not only insulting to the veterinary profession and your intelligence; it's also wrong.

There *are* conscientious dental technicians who are skilled at what they do. Certification is available as a "Master Dentist" to those who pass a rigorous set of qualifications. Such people will be happy to work with your veterinarian and not insult their profession.

There are other problems with teeth, like abscesses and infections.[5] Mercifully, they are not all that common. Removing an abscessed molar can be major surgery. The back teeth are so tightly packed together that they often cannot be removed from the mouth and they actually have to be driven out from the root side.

Care of your horse's teeth is the job of your veterinarian. Between your common sense and his or her good care, it's highly unlikely that your horse will ever have any major dental problems.

PART IV

WHEN THINGS GO WRONG

10

Colics

You've most likely had a colic. And, if you're a parent, your child has, too. Most likely the colics that you had as an infant weren't serious or you wouldn't be reading this book.

"Colic" is simply an old medical term. All it means is that there is pain coming from somewhere in the abdomen.[1] That's all it means in people. That's all it means in horses, too. It doesn't mean that something terrible is happening or that your horse is about to die. If your horse has a colic, it means that something inside hurts.

Let's say that you have a stomachache. Maybe it's because you made a pig out of yourself at the dinner table or maybe you had some bad chicken salad. Maybe you don't know why you feel so bad. If you just lie down (remember this and have sympathy for your horse), possibly take a bit of something and relax for a while, it will pass. Most of the time, when your stomach hurts, you'll be just fine.

Yet sometimes when your "stomach" hurts, it could be more serious than a simple stomachache. You could have appendicitis. If you have appendicitis, you need surgery. If you don't get your appendix removed, you're in big trouble. Fortunately, pain from your abdomen is usually not a serious problem.

Horses are the same way. Most of the time when a horse colics, it's not serious. He may be constipated or he may have some gas in his intestines. He may have a spasm in his gut or he may have eaten some bad feed. With some patience and possibly some medication, most colics will pass. Sometimes, however, the condition will be serious and require surgical intervention.

SIGNS

If your horse colics he will be uncomfortable. He will look back at his side. (The side he looks back at is not necessarily where the problem is.) He may stretch out. If your horse is male, he may act like he is having trouble urinating. He may paw or sweat. He may lie down and get up. He may roll around and thrash. His pain will not necessarily tell you how serious the colic is, but you will definitely know that something is wrong. The colicking horse will almost never have a fever. (If he does, it is almost always a sign that something else is going on besides just a "routine" colic caused by gas or impacted feed.)

When your horse colics, you will most likely be upset. You will be worried because you don't know if this is the end for your horse or not. You will see him in pain and you will want to do something, anything, to help.

Remember this: The vast majority of colicking horses do not need surgery. Most of them will pull through just fine.

Remember that and you won't panic. Veterinarians have a hard time talking to panic-stricken people. Don't panic and make it hard on your veterinarian, who already has his or her hands full with your horse.

THE DECISION FOR COLIC SURGERY

Ultimately, there is only one thing to decide about a colic in your horse. You and your veterinarian need to decide quickly if your horse needs to have surgery. That's it. If your horse doesn't need surgery, he will usually get better, even though he may require treatment. If your horse needs surgery, he needs to get to the hospital as soon as possible. The surgeon will then open up your horse's abdomen and straighten things out.

You do not want colic surgery to be a last resort. You want your horse to be as healthy as possible for surgery. Surgery puts stress on the horse's system, and a system that is as robust as possible is one that withstands stress the best. If your horse is about to die, surgery is a poor way to try to reverse the process. When death is coming, many irreversible changes in the horse's system begin to occur, and even the best surgeon can't reverse these changes.

There are dozens of problems that require surgical corrections. The type of surgical colic that your horse has is not important stall-side. It is only important to recognize that your horse's colic problem requires surgery as quickly as possible and to get him somewhere where it can be corrected immediately.

Colic surgeries are good things. That is, they are an effective way to keep your horse from dying from a surgical colic. Horse owners fear that after a colic surgery the horse will never come back to "what he was." If he needs colic surgery and doesn't get it, he will never come back at all! Horses are not permanently weakened after colic surgery. They generally *don't* have continual problems after surgery, although after surgery certain problems *can* occur. The potential problems with colic surgery should be explained to you at the time of surgery. Some of these complications can be quite serious; others can be handled relatively easily.[2]

Undoubtedly, you will meet someone whose horse did not do well after colic surgery. So many variables are involved with a successful outcome after surgery that it is impossible and imprudent to make generalizations about why things sometimes don't work out. However, if a surgical problem is recognized quickly, the horse is in good physical condition (not in shock) and he is operated on quickly, then the chances of a successful outcome are good.

If your horse has been diagnosed with some sort of a surgical problem, get him to a hospital. A twisted intestine will not correct itself. Also, a twisted intestine cannot be corrected by a routine rectal examination, so don't expect miracles from your vet in the field. Your veterinarian cannot reach into the horse's abdomen and straighten things out. For surgical colic problems, call a colic surgeon.

The trouble with colics is that it's not always easy, even if you're trained, to tell if a colic is medical (the type that goes away) or surgical (the type that can make the horse go away). There is much data to be collected about your horse to help make the decision.[3,4] If your horse has a colic, the best thing to do is to call your veterinarian. Let him or her decide if the problem is serious or not. Let him or her treat the horse. You should be ready to make observations about your horse's condition and response to treatment, stay in touch with your veterinarian and follow his or her advice. And be ready to go to surgery if you decide that is an option for your horse.

THE MYTHS ABOUT COLIC

People are curious animals. They want to know why things happen. They want to know how to fix the problem. They want to know how they can prevent a problem from happening again. And most of all, they want the problem to be the fault of somebody or something. It is in answer to these concerns that most of the myths about colics arise.

Just because people give you an answer doesn't mean that they know what they are talking about. Rarely does the fact that someone doesn't know stop him or her from pretending to know, either.

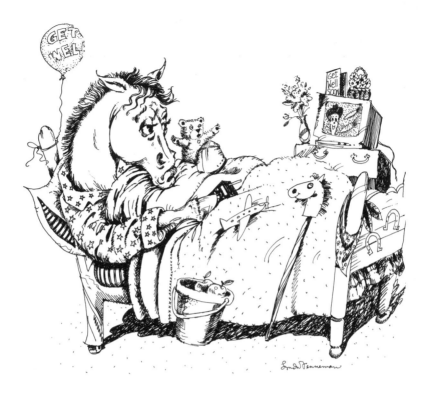

A horse with colic will not feel well.

WALKING THE COLICKING HORSE

One of the most common myths in the treatment of colics is the importance of walking the sick horse. Apparently, according to lore, walking the horse can either fix the colic or keep bad things from happening. It can't. However, some people feel that walking has a mild pain-relieving effect.[5]

There are a couple of variations on this "walking the colicking horse" theme. Some are even inadvertently humorous. For instance, you may hear, "As long as your horse keeps walking he won't be able to lie down and die." There is some sort of weird logic to this line of thinking, but in point of fact, if the horse does die, he will lie down.

If you insist on walking your colicking horse, at least be reasonable. The author has seen people beating poor, sick horses in an effort to keep them up and walking. Forcing the colicking horse to walk when he feels so bad is barbaric.

Look at it this way. Your stomach hurts. You lie down in front of the television. You start to feel better. Along comes your best friend and says "Okay, let's get up! Let's walk! Let's go!" This is justifiable grounds for homicide.

It's the same with your horse. He is down because he is uncomfortable. If he will lie quietly, let him lie there.

That being said, in the author's experience, sometimes, in very mild colics, a short amount of vigorous exercise (trot and canter at the longe for ten minutes) can relieve a horse's colic. Mild exercise may shake up a gas bubble or make the horse forget about his mild spasm.

You can sometimes see the same effect after a trailer ride to the hospital. You load your terribly sick horse on the trailer, drive like a maniac, elevate your blood pressure and arrive at the hospital to find your horse with his ears up and looking for something to eat. You will then find that even though the *colic* hasn't killed your horse, the stress of the whole situation will make *you* want to do it.

Whatever the reason, jostling the colicking horse about a little bit does seem to relieve colic pain on occasion. But if the pain persists after a brief bit of exercise (or a trailer ride), it's time to call your veterinarian.

ROLLING

Just as commonly, people are concerned about their horse rolling in the stall. Walking is a pretty good way to keep the horse from rolling. Not that rolling is much of a problem, of course. A common myth goes like this: "Don't let him roll, he may twist his gut." This just doesn't happen. Veterinarians don't know why horses' intestines twist.

Just because a horse rolls doesn't mean he's going to twist his gut. And just because his gut is twisted and he happened to roll doesn't mean that the rolling caused the twisting. In fact, horses roll all the time when they get turned out for exercise. They run around and roll around and they seem never to twist their guts doing this. It's not any different with a colic. Given the fact that there are a hundred feet or so of intestines in the abdomen and that it is arranged somewhat haphazardly, it is surprising that horses don't have more twisted intestines than they do!

Horses lie down and roll when they get colic because they are uncomfortable. They are trying to find a nice, comfortable place to lie down and be left alone (like a couch, in front of the television). The most serious colics, those with twisted intestines, are very painful for the horse. The horse with a twisted intestine rolls around a lot because the intestine is twisted, not the other way around.

The only problem that comes from rolling around is that the horse may scrape himself in a stall. If this is a problem, take the horse out of the stall to a bigger and softer area if you can. Keeping the horse from rolling doesn't do anything to treat a colic. Mostly, it gives the anxious owner something to do until the veterinarian arrives.

WEATHER CHANGES

The weather is frequently implicated as a cause of colics. A change of weather —if it's too cold, or hot, or wet, or dry—is sure to bring on a colic, right?

Well, believe it or not, there have been at least two studies trying to associate weather changes with the incidence of colics. The studies have related changes in barometric pressure (the most reliable indicator of changing weather) to the incidence of colic, and you know what? There's no apparent association between changing weather and incidence of colic.[6,7] Nor are there lunar, tidal or geologic influences.

PREVENTING COLIC

Frankly, most of the time, veterinarians don't know why a horse colics. Colic isn't a single disease process—in the same way that cancer is not a single disease. There are many causes of colic. Experimentally, the only practical way to *create* a colic is either to tie a string around the gut (to shut off the flow of blood and ingesta) or to blow up a balloon inside it. Obviously, neither of these models really is the same as a natural colic. No one knows why horse intestines twist, get out of place or impact with feed. The true initiating cause of most colics will most likely always remain a mystery. Since colic is such a dramatic and irritating problem, naturally folks would like to do whatever it takes to prevent it. This leads to a whole host of things that are done to "prevent" colics.

"PREVENTIVE" FEEDS

Feeding things (or not feeding things) to horses is a relatively popular way to prevent colic. Anything that is fed to a horse is moved on through the intestines relatively rapidly (since that's what intestines do). Once these things are out of the intestines, however, they have no residual effect at preventing a colic. So, unfortunately, no amount of daily bran, mineral oil or psyllium is going to ensure that your horse won't colic.

COLIC AND THE DIET

While on the subject of feeding, surely you've heard that it's very important not to make changes in the horse's diet too rapidly for fear of causing a colic. For instance, if you switch from alfalfa to a grass-type hay, it *must* be done over several days to prevent colic. Well, even though this is a commonly accepted practice, there's really no research to support it. Not that it hurts to change feed gradually; it just may not be all that important.

If a horse eats a lot of moldy hay, new grass or very green hay ("rich" hay), he may colic. Moldy hay or very green hay can make a horse feel awful. This type of feed can produce gas, which stretches the intestines and causes pain.[8] (Stretching the intestines is how the experimental balloon model causes pain.)

This type of colic is easy to help prevent. Check your hay or feed to make sure it's good quality and fresh before feeding it to your horse and don't let your horse overgraze fresh green pasture. Good hay smells good and it's green in color, as opposed to brown, musty and dusty. Why would you want to feed your buddy any other kind of hay?

You should probably feed your horse at regular intervals. In the wild, horses graze. They eat in a similar pattern to that of cats. Horses like to eat a little bit constantly.[9] People take horses and put them in boxes and feed them twice a day. For most of the day the horse is bored and starving. The rest of the day he is eating as rapidly as he can. Feeding several times a day will prolong the time that the horse takes to eat, mimic more closely the "natural" way of eating and help prevent boredom. *Maybe* regular feeding will also help decrease the incidence of colic, but there's no research to support that idea. If you can feed only twice a day, you probably should try to do it at the same times each day, just to keep a regular flow of ingested feed going through the horse. Clearly horses can exist just fine while being fed twice a day because most horses exist just this way. It's just that their system is designed otherwise.

BRAN

Can you prevent colic by feeding bran? In a word, no. Bran is made from wheat, and it is a very palatable source of protein and fiber for the horse. In the study of human nutrition, medicine has found that fiber is an effective way to help keep a person "regular" and that fiber is an important component of a good diet. It is difficult to imagine a diet with more fiber in it than that of the horse. Bran is a poor sister to hay when it comes to fiber.

So why is bran prescribed so much for colics? Why has it developed this mysterious reputation as curative of and preventive for colics? There are most likely several reasons, in the author's opinion. First of all, feeding bran to colicking horses has probably been done forever and no one has seen any real reason to stop (or has been bold enough to try). Just because bran really doesn't do anything for horses doesn't mean that well-meaning owners will stop using it. There must also be a feeling that if it's good for the owners, it *must* be good for their horses.

Seeing if a horse will eat bran does have some diagnostic value. Horses like to eat, and they particularly like to eat bran because it tastes good. Therefore, if a horse won't eat bran, especially after he has been given a pain-relieving drug, it is a sign that he doesn't feel very well at all. This bit of information is one more thing to use to help decide if the horse's problem is of a more serious nature. (Using the same logic, however, horses can also be fed sugar, apples, grass and carrots to see how serious a colic is.) Also, the mere presence of food in the intestine can be a stimulus for the intestine to move.[10,11] So if the horse eats bran (or anything else), it may stimulate some movement of the bowel. Getting the intestine to move may help push out the problem if the horse is impacted with feed or bloated with gas.

Bran is also a useful vehicle by which water can be put into a horse's system. A wet bran mash may be a limited way to help moisten a constipated mass of feed or help maintain his overall hydration as the water is absorbed by the bowel. Bran is *not* a laxative in horses, contrary to popular belief. Experimentally, diets high in bran have produced no noticeable change in the consistency of the horse's manure.[12] But horses do like the stuff.

VINEGAR

Vinegar in the diet as a "preventive" has some recent proponents. One of the causes of colic is the formation of intestinal stones. Some horses form stones (enteroliths) in their intestines, for reasons that no one knows. A stone forms much as a pearl forms in an oyster. Layer upon layer of material is deposited, sometimes around some intestinal irritant (like a piece of rope or a bottle cap) until a large stone forms. If the stone becomes large enough, it can block the intestine. When it does, the stone (or stones) has to be surgically removed.

The vinegar people believe a half cup of vinegar in the diet will prevent the formation of stones by "acidifying" the intestinal environment. Vinegar in the diet will make the intestinal environment more acid, but whether it actually prevents stone formation is anyone's guess. You can't hurt your horse by feeding him vinegar. Incidentally, many of the same people who promote the feeding of vinegar also say that feeding bran helps cause the stones.[13] There's no evidence to support either of these views at this time.

OTHER PREVENTIVES

What about other things to prevent colics? It has long been felt that horses that are heavily parasitized (lots of worms) may colic more often than horses that are kept relatively parasite free.[8] The solution to the parasite problem? Simple—deworm your horse regularly with an effective product.

As important as parasites are thought to be as a cause of colic, though, in a recent study of 229 horses with colic, there was no association with the deworming schedule or type of dewormer used and the history of colic. Most of these horses had all been dewormed regularly with effective products. Apparently, horses will colic whether or not they have been dewormed.[14]

SAND AND COLIC

Sand in the intestines is a known source of intestinal irritation and colic. Sand accumulates in the intestines of horses that like to pick up every little scrap of food from sandy ground. This type of horse will comb the ground for hours looking for that one alfalfa leaf. Along with the leaf of hay, he may also pick up several mouthfuls of sand. Over time, the sand can gather in the intestines.

One of the more common early signs of sand accumulation in the intestine (other than colic) is diarrhea. Sand in the bowel causes irritation to the intestinal lining. The intestines respond to any irritation by secreting water. Too much water in the manure is referred to as diarrhea.

But if too much sand accumulates in the intestines, it can create an obstruction. The sand can become a big blob of cement in the middle of the gut. Nothing can get by, everything stops up and pain begins.

If you live in an area where horses are kept in sandy corrals or pastures, you should check their manure frequently for sand. Simply take some fresh manure (from the top of the pile, so you don't pick up any extra sand) and mix it with water. Since the sand is heavier than anything else, it will end up on the bottom of the bucket. If there is a tablespoon of sand in a handful of manure, the horse should be treated to remove the sand.

There are a variety of products available to clean out sand from the intestines. They generally contain psyllium, the same stuff that's in fiber-based laxatives for people. It really seems to be the only thing that works very well in removing sand from a horse's intestines. Contrary to popular belief, wheat bran and mineral oil have not proven to be very effective at either preventing or treating sand accumulation in the horse's bowel.[15]

MEDICAL TREATMENT OF COLIC

Medical treatment of colics is aimed at just two things: controlling the horse's pain and helping correct the internal problems. All colics are painful (if your horse wasn't hurting you wouldn't know there was a colic). Pain itself causes the intestines to slow down, so in addition to humane reasons for controlling the colicking horse's pain, there are medical considerations for pain relief as well. There are many pain-relieving drugs out there, and which one (or ones) is used is frequently based on the experience of the attending veterinarian. In addition, the horse's response to pain-relieving drugs can be a useful indicator of whether or not there is a serious problem.

Veterinarians attempt to correct the cause of a colic that is amenable to medical treatment by putting things into the horse's system that relieve gas or help push through an obstruction. Most commonly, light mineral oil is given via a tube that is passed through the nose into the stomach. Mineral oil is a very mild laxative. While many people think that mineral oil lubricates the intestines, some of its effects may be that it interferes with the absorption of water in the intestine. When trying to soften a mass of manure, the more water in the intestines, the better. Mineral oil doesn't penetrate what's in the intestines well, and so it most likely softens the manure very little if at all. Mineral oil works best at helping pass manure that has already been dislodged from an impaction.[16]

There are other substances, such as Epsom salts and dioctyl sodium sulfosuccinate (called DSS, for obvious reasons), that can be given to a colicking horse as well, depending on your vet's preference. Epsom salts (magnesium sulfate) draws water into the bowel and can be useful in helping break up an impacted mass. Always give Epsom salts with water to avoid intestinal irritation.

DSS has all sorts of good effects. It softens manure by allowing water to penetrate it. It also increases fluid secretion into the bowel, and in high doses it can even stimulate intestinal movement.[16,17]

Horses with a medical colic generally get better with treatment. No medication is going to fix a horse with a surgical problem. There's certainly no best medication to give to all horses with colic.

DEHYDRATION

Another medical consideration in colic therapy is the horse's state of hydration. In addition to metabolic reasons for dehydration (which are complicated), many colicking horses won't drink because they hurt and won't take in enough water to support themselves. This can become a problem.

Very commonly, people will perform a simple test to see if the horse is dehydrated. They will take a pinch of skin from the neck and see if it "stands up," that is, see if the skin returns to its normal contour quickly. If it doesn't, people assume that the horse is dehydrated.

Unfortunately, the pinch test is not nearly as accurate as people would like it to be. The presence of a standing skin fold after a pinch does not necessarily mean that a horse is getting dehydrated. It may only mean that the skin is sort of loose in the area that was pinched. The first signs of dehydration are subtle. Your veterinarian will recognize the signs of dehydration in your horse and proceed to correct them accordingly if necessary. If your horse is significantly dehydrated, aggressive treatment measures such as the administration of intravenous fluids may be required in medical management of a colicking horse.

Unfortunately, in spite of your best management efforts, horses are going to colic from time to time. If your horse colics, it is most likely not your fault (or anyone else's). The diagnosis and treatment of a colic is best left to your veterinarian. Collection and interpretation of a variety of clinical signs is important for rapid and accurate diagnosis. Like everything else that you will read in this book, the best approach to a colic is the level-headed one: Recognize the problem and get some help. And don't believe everything you hear.

11

Strangles

There is a bacterial respiratory disease that bothers horses and really bothers their owners. Innocently enough, it is caused by *Streptococcus*, the same bacteria that cause strep throat in people. To the never-ending dismay of horse owners, this disease has been given the frightful and awe-inspiring name of strangles.

It's likely that nearly everything you've heard about strangles is wrong. You'll feel better about this disease after you've read this chapter.

The strangles bacteria enter the nasal passages and attach to the lymph nodes of the pharynx (the area at the back of the throat where the oral and nasal passages meet). The bacteria happily and speedily reproduce there and then spread to other lymph nodes, particularly those under the jaw (submandibular lymph nodes). There, the lymph nodes try to fight off the bacteria. As a result, an abscess forms.

SIGNS

The first signs of strangles that you will notice are fever and lethargy. The horse generally won't eat. Pretty soon, the horse's nose will look like it is packed with mayonnaise. Within a few days or weeks the lymph nodes under the jaw will abscess and rupture, releasing lots of pus and goo. Then the abscess heals and the horse is fine. The whole messy ordeal usually takes a couple of weeks.

That's it. Sure, complications can arise. Horses can die from strangles, but they very rarely do. Horses die from the flu. Although the disease can be a nuisance in a young herd of horses (and a mess to clean up), it is generally not a serious health risk to the horse, at least in terms of any long-term consequences. Probably the name of the disease, "strangles," is responsible for the sort of mass hysteria the disease induces in owners.

It is an awful name.

As the disease develops, the swelling of the lymph nodes under the jaw can get quite dramatic. The swelling has the *potential* to impede the passage of air through the windpipe. But this is quite unusual. Some horses experience difficulty in breathing if the swelling gets too bad. They are effectively "strangled" by the swelling. Ideally, you will take care of the situation long before it reaches this point.

Just because a horse has a swelling under the jaw doesn't mean he has strangles. If he doesn't have any of the other signs of strangles, the swelling is probably caused by something else.

CONTROLLING THE DISEASE

Strangles requires direct contact, either with infected horses or contaminated surfaces, for the disease to spread.[1] That is, for the bacteria to go from horse to horse, infected horses must be in direct contact with either each other or with contaminated things like feed buckets or waterers. Flies are said to be able to carry the disease, too, but there have been no studies to show that they do.

Viral diseases such as flu and rhino are easily spread through aerosol droplets that get coughed and sneezed out by a sick horse. They can spread through the air and move through a barn quite rapidly. Strangles, however, has a bit more difficulty moving from horse to horse unless the horses are kept together. In a pasture full of yearlings, where everybody shares feeders and waterers and rubs noses, the disease can move rapidly. However, a box stall is a very effective barrier to the spread of strangles.

Therefore, to control this disease, it is very important to remove and isolate infected horses from the healthy ones. Feeders and waterers and stall walls must be kept especially clean and disinfected because the bacteria can live for a while on surfaces.[2] But while it is very important to keep healthy horses away from the sick ones, what appears not to be very important is to vaccinate the herd against the disease.

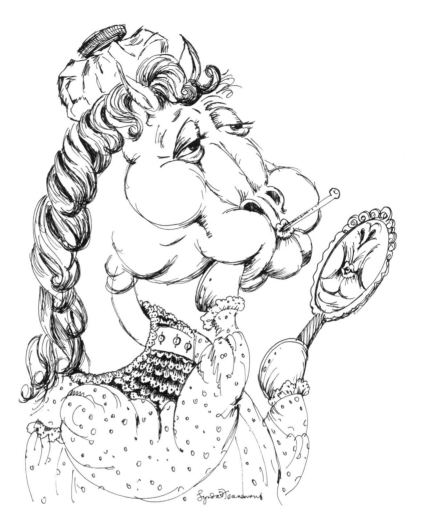

Swelling of the face is a typical sign of strangles.

STRANGLES AND VACCINATION

It would be great if there were a really effective vaccine against strangles. Vaccines are wonderful things. An effective vaccine is invented and bang, no more polio. Not all diseases are as amenable to being eliminated, however. For instance, there is no effective vaccine against colds in humans. With strangles, the most optimistic study ever done showed an approximately 50 percent protection rate at preventing the strangles infection (using one of the available vaccines), in a group of horses kept together in very tight quarters.[3] You could argue that 50 percent protection is better than nothing. You can't argue, however, that isolation of infected horses and disinfection of contaminated areas and items such as brushes and halters are the most effective things that you can do to prevent the spread of strangles.

Apparently, the reason that the strangles vaccine doesn't work very well is that although it produces a good level of immune factors (antibodies) in the blood, immune factors in the blood aren't very important in fighting off the disease. Even if blood immune levels are high, the vaccines don't produce immunity in the tissues of the pharynx, the site where the bacteria attach. When it comes to preventing this disease, local immunity in the pharynx is evidently much more important than the circulating immune factors in the blood.[4] Veterinarians are waiting for a vaccine that creates a high immune level where it's needed.

Vaccination of healthy horses is not without problems of its own. The strangles vaccine is reported to be one of the more common vaccines that causes local tissue reaction. Swelling in the injection site, abscesses and local scarring are all things that have been reported as a result of the strangles vaccine.[1,2] Although these problems can occur with any vaccine, in the author's experience they occur more frequently with the strangles vaccine.

If you have horses that are *sick* with strangles, at least you should vaccinate them and all the other horses, to try and control the spread, right? Big myth. There is a big problem associated with vaccination in the face of a strangles outbreak: an adverse immune reaction called purpura hemorrhagica (yes, it is really called that). Purpura is an inflammation of the blood vessels, the result of a reaction between the blood vessels and immune factors. It can occur as a result of infection or as a result of the immune system stimulation that can occur, though rarely, from a single vaccination.

Horses can develop purpura "naturally" several weeks after recovering from respiratory disease.[5] But it has also been shown that vaccinating sick horses or horses harboring disease in its early stages can increase the chances of the horse getting this reaction.[1]

The signs of purpura are unmistakable. The whole horse swells up. His legs swell and his face swells. He feels miserable and looks worse. The disease can be fatal, though it's usually not. A horse in this state needs aggressive treatment.

STRANGLES AND PENICILLIN

What about treating the horses?

Here's some good news. It's another myth breaker, however. Penicillin is a great drug that can help prevent or treat strangles. The *Streptococcus* bacteria that cause this disease have not yet developed a resistance to penicillin. Lots of bacteria, after being exposed to an antibiotic, become resistant to it, which can be a real problem in some infections. Antibiotic resistance by bacteria is one of the reasons that researchers and drug companies are always trying to invent new and more powerful antibiotics. Perhaps the strangles bacteria is slow. Whatever the reason, and fortunately for horses, the bacteria are almost always killed effectively by penicillin.[2]

Even so, penicillin should be used judiciously and sensibly in the treatment of strangles. If your horse has already developed an abscess under his jaw, penicillin will tend to delay the opening of the abscess.[2] An abscess is a mass of pus with a thick wall of inflamed tissue around it. It's very difficult for antibiotics to penetrate into this gooey mess of bacteria, white blood cells and tissue debris. Giving penicillin to a horse with an abscess tends to slow down an abscess by killing the most easily reached bacteria on the fringes of the abscess. It can't cause the pus to be removed or absorbed. It's usually easier to let the abscess rupture (or cut it open) and then start the horse on penicillin to kill off any remaining bacteria while the abscess heals.

Penicillin, however, can be very effective at treating strangles if it is given before an abscess forms.[2] You can kill the bacteria before they make a big mess of your horse's jaw. If your horse is in the middle of a strangles outbreak, you should monitor his temperature very closely and begin treatment with penicillin if he stops eating or develops either a nasal discharge or a fever.

You can even give penicillin to healthy horses in the face of a disease outbreak.[2] Prophylactic (preventive) use of penicillin is pretty effective at helping to control the spread of the disease, in conjunction with isolation and disinfection.

"But wait!" you cry. "Penicillin can drive the infection into the body and cause abscesses of the internal lymph nodes, right? Using penicillin to treat horses with strangles is bad, right?"

Oh, sigh.

In some horses (very few), the abscesses do occur in places besides the lymph nodes under the jaw. Since this complication is particularly horrible, it has been given the particularly horrible name of "bastard" strangles. Sometimes strangles abscesses just seem to keep popping up at various spots on the horse's body. As long as the abscesses keep rupturing to the outside, however, the horse will be fine in time, though quite miserable to be around (and messy!) until all of the abscesses have stopped forming. But if abscesses occur in the abdominal lymph nodes and bacteria rupture into the abdomen, for example, the consequences can be fatal. Horses can recover if the abscesses are caught in time.[1,2]

Penicillin has gotten an undeserved reputation in the treatment of strangles. In 1972 a book for medical doctors discussed the current thoughts on streptococcal diseases. (This is not light reading, and it is not out in paperback.) The editors invited a couple of veterinarians to write a chapter for their book. These two veterinarians said, "Clinical observations suggest that bastard strangles occurs more frequently when horses with immature abscesses are treated with penicillin than in individuals not so treated. These observations support the view that the development of the disseminated, more chronic form of the disease may be due to an effect of penicillin on the organism."[6]

That's it. Two guys thought this *might* happen.

Mind you, there was nothing cited in the paper to support this observation.

This paper has been referenced and passed on ever since 1972, and you find lots of veterinarians and horse people who believe it. There is absolutely no experimental evidence to support this idea of driving bacteria to hide inside the horse's body. In fact, if the horse does develop abscesses of the internal lymph nodes, guess how you treat him. With high doses of penicillin, of course!

POST-STRANGLES IMMUNITY

One last myth to kill. Many people believe that after a horse has strangles once he can never get it again. There is no lifelong immunity to strangles obtained by getting the disease. Your horse can get strangles again if he's had it before. Naturally occurring immunity lasts for six to twelve months.[1,2]

Good management techniques are the best way to control and prevent strangles in horses. New arrivals should be isolated for up to thirty days, if possible, to help prevent the introduction of strangles (or any other new disease) onto your premises. Sick horses should be removed from an infected herd and all animals in the herd should be monitored closely for early signs of infection, such as fever, so that they can be treated quickly, prior to the development of abscesses. If you do choose to vaccinate your horses, realize that the vaccines do not provide very effective protection and have the potential to cause side effects.

Although control of strangles may be time consuming and tedious, it can be effectively done. This is not a killer disease. There's really nothing to be afraid of.

12

Wounds

It has been said that horses are creatures bent on committing suicide, looking only for an inappropriate and inconvenient place to pull it off. As such, they get to cut themselves a lot, probably just to see what it feels like in preparation for the big event.

Horses find the most insignificant little things to cut themselves on. The big things must be obvious to them. Turn a horse out in a field full of rusted barbed wire and old nails and usually he will be just fine. However, if the head of a screw is sticking out from the wall of a stall by one eighth of an inch, it seems like a horse will sustain a major laceration right away.

How horses cut themselves can be quite mysterious. Sometimes there is a telltale bit of hair or blood on a sharp corner. Other times you will be unable to find even the least bit of evidence as to what caused the huge gash on your horse's side. The author's personal conviction is that horses rarely actually "cut" themselves. Rather, they walk by a threatening-looking bit of material and their skin sort of spontaneously springs open.

Seriously, though, horses do seem to cut themselves with alarming frequency. What is many times even more alarming is the response of the owner. Wounds should always be handled in a careful, well-thought-out, level-headed manner.

Wounds behave in a very predictable fashion. You can anticipate a lot about what is going to happen with a healing wound. With the exception of the most dramatic ones, wounds are rarely threatening to life or limb.

The first thing you should do if your horse has a cut is try to make some sort of a rational assessment as to how serious the wound is. Please note the word "rational." Phrases like "Oh my God, it's horrible" are rarely helpful or appropriate, especially when used to describe a wound that is almost imperceptible. Take time to examine the wound. When you have reached some sort of conclusion (for instance, that the wound is two inches long and not very deep and on the front part of the leg), you will then be able to communicate what the problem is to your veterinarian. Your veterinarian will advise you what to do until he or she is able to attend to your horse. This sort of dispassionate look at a wound is important as well for your state of mind.

TREATING MINOR WOUNDS

The skin is a barrier to the outside. If this barrier is not penetrated or disrupted by a wound, nothing bad is going to happen to the horse. Minor scrapes happen all the time and are almost never anything to worry about. The author's experience is that many people worry more about wounds on their horse than those on themselves. Minor scrapes, while occasionally quite traumatic for the owner, are the equivalent of a close shave (literally) for the horse. Even if this type of wound develops a slightly reddened appearance, from the removal of a few superficial skin cells, it is virtually impossible to mess the wound up by providing treatment. It makes absolutely no difference what you do to or for these superficial scrapes (within humane constraints, of course).

After your horse scrapes himself, legions of people will descend on your stall with advice and suggestions about what you must do to cure your horse's minor abrasion. For scrapes, most likely anything and everything will work. You can apply almost any sort of wound dressing or bandage, in one of a wide variety of colors (both bandage and dressing), to these minor wounds with a successful end result. Of course, if you do nothing at all, your horse will be fine, too.

TREATING DEEPER WOUNDS

Deeper wounds require more care and a more thoughtful approach than do minor scrapes. Two things will give you a clue as to whether or not a wound is deep. First, you will most likely see blood. Second, you may see the stuff that's supposed to be under the skin. Skin is supposed to keep the outsides out and the insides in. Cuts disrupt this important function. While either of these circumstances may be somewhat disconcerting to you, even in the most serious wounds, they demand a rational approach.

Flowing blood comes from cut blood vessels. Bigger vessels bleed more. Arteries tend to spurt when cut. (This is because they have blood in them that is being moved under pressure from the pumping of the heart.) It really doesn't matter what kind of blood your horse is losing in a cut, only that you recognize that your horse is bleeding (which generally isn't hard to do). You will then want to take steps to stop the bleeding.

STOPPING THE BLEEDING

From a medical standpoint, cut and bleeding horses are great patients because they have so darn much blood. Blood loss can be critical in some patients. In canaries, for instance, the loss of a couple of drops can be fatal. In horses, the loss of a couple of *buckets* is not a big deal, since most adult horses have nine or ten gallons. Blood clots more slowly in horses than in other species, and the fifteen or so minutes[1] that it may take for blood to stop flowing in a cut horse can seem like forever.

The obvious thing to do about the blood exiting from a wound is to try to stop it from coming out. This requires the application of pressure in some form, be it by a bandage or your hand. What you use to apply pressure with is not particularly important, and any number of relatively clean rags, bandages or articles of clothing will suffice. Don't fuss too much over what to use to stop bleeding.

While it may be terribly tempting to use a tourniquet on a cut horse, don't do it. Direct pressure is almost always the best way to stop bleeding. You can do much more harm than good with a poorly applied tourniquet, and horses tend to resent them because of the pressure tourniquets apply to the leg. While trying to help your horse, you could get yourself kicked.

CLEANING THE WOUND

After the bleeding has stopped, you have to deal with the stuff that's under the skin. If you see the stuff that's under the skin, cover it up. It's not meant to see the light of day. At the time of the injury, it doesn't matter to you (or the horse, for that matter) what the cut has exposed. You are not going to be able to do anything to fix the problem, anyway. Your job is to keep dirt out of the wound so that it can eventually be repaired by your veterinarian.

Cleaning and scrubbing a fresh wound is not as important as you would think. If the wound is packed with dirt and gravel, it's a good idea to try to get most of the dirt out of the wound by rinsing it with water or something. But incessant rubbing and watering of a wound can retard blood clotting, since it washes away the little clots that are trying to form on the blood vessels. Too much water on tissue isn't good for the tissue, either. Water is quite different from the fluid that makes up the body (the body fluid has a lot of salts in it and water doesn't). Exposed tissue absorbs water, and water causes exposed tissue to swell and look gray and waterlogged.[2] A good quick rinse to remove the big chunks of contaminating material is great, but leave the thorough cleaning to your veterinarian, who is going to have to repair the wound.

What sort of solution you use for the initial cleaning is certainly not very important. Horse owners will run around frantically looking for a tamed iodine solution or hydrogen peroxide while the horse stands there patiently with a bleeding, dirty wound. (Hydrogen peroxide is generally *not* recommended for the treatment of fresh wounds, for a variety of reasons that have to do with its damaging effects on the tissue and small blood vessels.)[3] When cleaning a wound, carefully remove the large, obvious bits of material with a minimum of trauma to the wound and a minimum of hassle to yourself and the horse.

DRESSING THE WOUND

It's also not necessary to put a dressing on a fresh wound. A clean bandage will keep dirt out, and that's the most important thing. If you do put a dressing on a fresh wound, make sure that it is not one that will harm the tissue. Many over-the-counter wound products will do more harm than good to an open wound. One of them, for instance, is largely composed of carbonated lime, the same caustic stuff that you throw on the bottom of your horse's stall to help dry it up. This is not what you want on a fresh wound. It has been said that you should never put anything into a wound that you wouldn't put in your own eye!

After you have gently cleaned the wound, stopped the bleeding and put a clean bandage over the area (where possible), you should get your veterinarian involved in the repair of the wound.

WOUND REPAIR

Skin wounds can only repair themselves in one of two ways: first intention healing and second intention healing. First intention healing is the simplest, quickest and strongest way that a wound can heal and from a cosmetic point of view, the most desirable.

First Intention Healing

The best example of this type of healing is a surgical wound. A cut is made, stitches are placed on either side of the wound to bring the skin edges back together, the skin edges grow into each other and the wound is healed. As an added benefit with horses, the hair grows back over the wounded edges so you often will not even notice the scar from the wound that was there.

If you follow all of the principles of first aid that have been discussed and get your veterinarian to your horse as soon as possible, you have a good chance of this type of healing taking place. Although not all wounds can or should be handled by stitching them closed (a deep puncture, for instance, may be better left unsutured), those that can be immediately sewn up stand the best chance of healing rapidly, with normal function and appearance.

You have a limited amount of time to act if you expect a successful repair of a wound by first intention healing. This is referred to as the "golden period" in which wound repair is possible. If your horse cuts himself at eight o'clock at night, it may not be possible to repair the wound if you wait until eight o'clock the next morning. Veterinarians may grumble about having to come out at night to repair the wound, but in their hearts they know they're doing the right thing.

The golden period during which a wound can be successfully repaired primarily reflects the difference between two medical terms: contamination and infection. Your skin is contaminated. Bacteria are living all over it. Your skin is not infected. Infection occurs when bacteria penetrate deep into the tissue and start to grow.

When a cut occurs, bacteria that have gotten under your horse's skin (literally) are living on the surface of the newly exposed subcutaneous tissue. The new wound is contaminated, just like the skin surface. The bacteria, however, have not yet had time to get beyond the surface of the wounded tissue. As such, your veterinarian can be fairly effective at removing them by cleansing and rinsing the wound. Once the bacteria are removed, the wound can be closed up so that the healing process can begin.

There is no hard and fast rule as to how long the golden period is. It depends on many factors, like the blood supply to the injured area, how bad the injury is, how contaminated the wound is and where on the horse the injury is located. Wounds of the face, for instance, can often be sutured even after a delay of twenty-four hours. Most leg wounds, however, need to be attended to within a couple of hours.[4] The bottom line? If your horse cuts himself, get your veterinarian there as soon as possible!

After the golden period expires, the bacteria will have had time to penetrate more deeply into the wound. At this point, the wound is said to be infected. This is a problem because no amount of scrubbing can remove an infection. It will be up to the body (possibly with an assist from some antibiotics) to get the infection under control before the wound can begin to heal.

Getting a wound infection under control can take several days. If the wound is closed prior to the infection being resolved, the closed wound will open up. The body cannot (and absolutely refuses to) heal over an infected area. The process of infection has a number of effects that prevent cells that are trying to heal the wound from doing so.[5] The best way of dealing with a wound infection is to prevent it, by good, sensible early wound care.

So to review what to do when confronted with a fresh wound: (1) stop the bleeding; (2) clean and cover the wound; and (3) get your veterinarian there fairly quickly. Nothing else really matters.

Second Intention Healing

Second intention healing generally gives horse owners fits. It occurs when the skin edges cannot be brought together.

If a wound is too old to be sutured or if the amount of tissue lost in the wound is too extensive, it may not be possible (at least immediately) to sew it back together. The horse's body will then go through a series of well-documented steps in an attempt to get the wound healed, that is, to get the insides covered up again. The body *always* tries to heal injured tissue (it's one of the rules of live tissue). The body is going to try to heal every wound unless something happens to stop it from doing so.

When the skin edges remain apart and unsutured, the wound will initially become infected, generally temporarily. Infection does not mean that the horse is going to lose his leg or that there will be a lot of swelling and pain. Infections can be very localized and almost imperceptible. That being said, the first thing that the body has to do on the way to healing its wound by second intention is to get rid of the infection. Unless the problem becomes more extensive, the horse is usually able to handle infection at the local level in four or five days. Sometimes it may be advisable to assist the body by providing it with antibiotics to kill or limit the growth of the bacteria in the wound. But once the bacteria are taken care of, the wound will begin to fill up with granulation tissue.

Granulation tissue is nothing to worry about. Its appearance on the scene is a good thing. It means that the body is starting to heal normally. Granulation tissue is produced to fill up the wound and begins to show up in a wound three to six days after the initial injury. This tissue is composed of collagen, one of the proteins that makes up tissue, and little blood vessels called capillaries.[6] That's it. No nerves, no hair follicles, no sweat glands. This is simple stuff.

Granulation tissue is also a virtually impenetrable barrier to infection. The huge concentration of blood vessels in granulation tissue means that bacteria are confronted with an aggressive front line of blood cells that fight infection. Bacteria can live on the surface of granulation tissue but have a terrible time living in it.[7]

You can do almost anything to a wound that has granulation tissue in it and the wound will not get infected. You can put onto granulation tissue any number of ointments and sprays and substances that are good to tissue and substances that are hard on tissue. In spite of your "treatment," granulation tissue will still try to form because it is *necessary* so that the wound can heal. Since you can do almost anything to granulation tissue and get away with it, almost everything is done to granulation tissue.

So to review quickly, in second intention healing the wound cannot be sutured, gets a little bit infected and once the infection is controlled, begins to grow a layer of helpful granulation tissue. The wound continues to heal. At this point, however, you may be able to do something else to speed up the healing process.

Delayed First Intention Healing

Four or five days after the occurrence of a wound, a good veterinarian may be able to play a trick on the body and get the wound to close by a technique known as delayed first intention healing. This is a very useful technique. It takes advantage of the fact that the body has cleaned up the infection and laid down tissue that cannot be infected over the top of the underlying tissue.

To close a wound with delayed technique, the veterinarian is basically creating a fresh wound from the old one. The five-day-old wound is prepared and scrubbed and the granulation tissue is removed, usually with a scalpel. This removes the surface debris and reveals healthy, uninfected tissue below. The new edges of the wound can then be brought together, and, happily reunited, they can grow together, just as if the wound had been sutured in the first place. This technique can be especially useful in treating wounds that happened in the middle of the night that never had an opportunity for first intention healing.[8]

Of course, not all wounds can be handled with a delayed closure technique. Some must be left to close by second intention. For instance, wounds on the lower leg that are accompanied by lots of tissue loss can be a real problem because horses have absolutely no extra skin in this area. In dogs (say, a slightly overweight Golden Retriever), there is often enough skin to make another dog. If these dogs lose a little skin, a veterinarian can just pull some more on over to cover up the area. In the lower leg of the horse, there is barely enough skin to cover what's there, much less make up for any that's lost due to injury. As a wound undergoing healing by second intention fills up with granulation tissue, the skin cells on the edges of the wound begin to reproduce. Ultimately, the cells on the edges intend to re-create the skin's barrier to the outside. In the healing second intention wound, you can notice a pink rim all around the wound edge made up of these rapidly growing cells. After four to six weeks, depending on the size of the wound, the granulation tissue will begin to contract and become smaller. Eventually, the new skin cells will unite and cover up the granulation tissue. At this point, the wound will be healed.[4,9]

In smaller wounds, second intention healing usually takes several weeks. In large wounds, this process of granulation tissue formation, contraction and growth of tissue from the edges of the wound (called epithelialization) can take many months before full wound coverage is achieved.

GRANULATION TISSUE

Two things about second intention healing seem to really bother horse people: the granulation tissue itself and the scar that results from this type of healing.

Granulation tissue first. People worry that a wound that is not sutured will develop proud flesh. This is another one of those colorful (and quite useless) horse terms. Proud flesh describes granulation tissue that has grown beyond the surface of the wound. Once beyond the wound surface, granulation tissue can proliferate and look ugly. Proud flesh is not abnormal tissue, however. It is normal tissue that has been allowed to overgrow. It is not "bad" for a wound. It is not dangerous to the horse. Its presence does not mean that your horse will be disfigured. It may mean that you haven't been paying enough attention to the wound, since there's no reason why a wound that has been attended to should form excessive granulation tissue.

Proud flesh commonly forms in large wounds that have a lot of area to be covered by the ingrowth of the cells from the sides of the wound. In large wounds, healing becomes a race to see if the cells will cover the granulation tissue before the granulation tissue grows beyond the edge of the wound and takes off.

Even though granulation tissue is not bad and never abnormal, it is occasionally necessary to control its growth so that a wound can heal. There are right ways to do this. There are wrong ways to do this. Do the right thing.

Granulation tissue growth is limited by what is called contact inhibition. That is, granulation tissue cells won't grow well if there is pressure against the growing cells, be it from contact with a neighboring cell on the side or from a bandage applied on the top. Therefore, one of the good ways to control granulation tissue is to inhibit its growth by direct contact with a bandage that applies slight pressure to the healing area.

The growth of granulation tissue can be also controlled by the use of corticosteroid-based ointments. These ointments slow the growth of granulation tissue when they are applied to the surface of the tissue. Happily, when applied starting five days from the initial injury, corticosteroid ointments do not also slow down the epithelial cells growing in from the sides of the wound.

Excessive granulation tissue also can be cut back with a scalpel. This can generally be done on a standing horse and without the use of local anesthetic because the granulation tissue has no nerves. It's quick and very effective (and dramatic), and well tolerated by the horse. Removing granulation tissue in this fashion is a bit bloody, since so much of granulation tissue is made up of blood vessels. Once the exuberant tissue has been removed and the bleeding has stopped, however, you will be astounded at how quickly the wound will look healthy.[9]

What you should not do to granulation tissue is put substances on it that are caustic and damaging to fresh tissue. Things like lime, kerosene, copper sulfate, pine tar or silver nitrate are awful things to put on fresh tissue. (If you put them in your eye, you'd go blind.) Remember, granulation tissue is normal, healing tissue. You don't want to damage it because it is trying to heal your horse. If you put caustic chemicals on the tissue you will induce a chemical burn. The body will not heal over this newly damaged tissue until the damaged tissue itself has had time to heal. By damaging the wound with these chemicals you can delay healing.[9] Throw away those powders and sprays. Stop burning your horse's granulation tissue!

There are sprays that are made up of enzymes that can be applied to granulation tissue. These enzymes are similar to those that are found in commercially available meat tenderizers. They do the same thing to the wound that the meat tenderizer does to your steak, that is, they digest protein. Enzymes do a good job of keeping granulation tissue clean and healthy. The surface proteins digested by them include bacterial debris and dead tissue of the wound. This allows for a cleaner, healthier surface of granulation tissue.[10]

You may have heard that putting meat tenderizer on granulation tissue is an effective way to control its growth. Well, it is. Meat tenderizer is made up of enzymes (and salt) and it actually works fairly well.

Eventually, granulation tissue will stop trying to proliferate. At this time, the tissue is mature. The time for tissue maturation can be quite variable, however; once it occurs, you won't have anything else to worry about, unless the tissue gets injured again and starts to regrow.

With granulation tissue, first find out if it needs to be controlled, and if it does, control it in a way that won't harm tissue. The wound will heal more quickly, and with less trouble, than if you try to take care of it in a misguided or poorly directed fashion.

SCAR TISSUE

The second thing that people worry about with second intention healing is the formation of a scar. A scar is composed of the mature cells that grow from the sides of a healing wound, over the granulation tissue. The cells that grow from the sides of the wound to cover it are not, unfortunately, the only cells that make up normal skin. Therefore, the covering that results from the growth of these cells doesn't have things like hair follicles, sweat glands or oil glands that are found in normal skin. The resulting healed tissue is kind of dry and crusty and it looks like, well, a big scar.

The best way to control scarring is by following the proper principles of wound care and getting the wound to close by first intention or delayed first intention healing. If a wound is too large to be handled in this way, a scar will be the inevitable result.

Large wounds of the neck, chest, body and upper legs tend to heal very nicely by second intention, with minimal scarring, even though they look kind of ugly while they are trying to heal. Usually a good, cosmetic end result is attained with these types of wounds. The biggest problems with scarring occur in the healing of wounds of the lower leg, where there is tissue loss and no extra skin to pull over to cover up the area.

With people who have a large wound of the lower limb with much skin loss, doctors use skin grafting to cover the affected area. Unfortunately, skin grafting is pretty tricky in the horse. But it is something that you can try so as to get large wounds covered and healed more quickly than would occur with normal healing. Plastic and reconstructive surgery may also help reduce the size of a scar in particular situations.[11]

You cannot make a scar grow hair because there are no hair follicles in scar tissue. You can't make *anything* grow hair, and if you could there would be legions of bald men who would be forever in your debt. So if people tell you that cold water, or cod liver oil, or vitamin E, or bacon grease or anything else can grow hair when it is put onto a wound, you should look at them with a bemused smile. You can try whatever they recommend, just don't pay them for it.

Bandages

Finally, a word about bandages. Bandages are very important tools in wound management. In fresh wounds, bandages are useful in controlling bleeding and in keeping the wound clean. In the treatment of healing wounds, bandages keep wounds clean, help control swelling (due to the counterpressure) and help absorb and remove wound fluids.

Additionally, in wounds that are subject to motion, such as those on the surface of the hock or the fetlock, bandages can be very important in reducing wound motion. Wounds have a terrible time healing across a moving surface, and a bandage can help immobilize an area. Sometimes it is even advisable to put a cast (which is just a rigid bandage) on a wound to control the motion of a healing wound. This is something that your veterinarian, not you, will be doing.

Application of a wound dressing under the bandage is usually a good idea in open wounds that are healing by second intention. Wound dressings can help control the growth of surface bacteria. The dressing should be applied on a nonstick pad so you don't rip off the surface of the healing wound each time you change the bandage.[12]

In sutured wounds, however, a wound dressing may not be all that important. Many surgeons feel that a sutured wound doesn't need to be covered with *any* type of dressing, as long as it is protected from additional trauma or contamination.[13] This is just one more thing to think about when someone starts telling you about all the stuff that you *have* to put on your horse's repaired wound.

Remember two simple things about wounds. First, all wounds will try to heal. Second, if they are not healing, something is wrong. A nonhealing wound should not be left alone; don't assume that it will heal eventually. Something keeps a nonhealing wound from closing, and your veterinarian just has to figure out what it is. Many complex factors are involved in wound healing. It is important to know about them and manage them so that good results can be obtained. Your veterinarian should be well versed in these factors, and his or her advice should be that which you are following. The experience of your friends will usually be based on one or two horses and no study; accept their advice graciously but pay it little heed.

Almost all wounds will heal if they are handled properly. Just because you want to do *something* to help your horse with a cut doesn't mean that you should do just *anything*. If you act rationally and on good advice you can usually count on a successful outcome for your horse's wound.

PART V

THE
MUSCULOSKELETAL
SYSTEM

13

Legs

Lots of things happen to horses' legs. Left to their own devices, horses take care of their legs pretty well. Of course, people jump horses over fences, run them around in circles, try to make them "rounder" and in short make them do all sorts of things they would just as soon not do. Inevitably things happen to horses' legs since they take so much abuse.

When there is a problem with the legs, the signs tend to be straightforward. You will immediately notice that your horse has a leg problem because of one of two things (or both). There will be a swelling on the leg or the horse will limp. That's about it.

LAMENESS

When a horse limps, he is said to be lame. The diagnosis of lameness is both an art and a science, and a lot of observation and inspection goes into a thorough and accurate examination for lameness.

It's a myth that you can always find out *why* a horse is lame. Unfortunately, even with advances in diagnostic equipment, some causes of lameness cannot be diagnosed. In the hoof, for example, veterinarians cannot distinguish between all the important ligaments and tendons by *any* available method. As a result, a veterinarian may be able to tell where your horse is lame but not necessarily why or exactly what is causing the problem.

Sometimes the location of the problem that causes a horse's lameness can be quite obvious. It doesn't require a great deal of diagnostic skill to see the nail that the horse stepped on is causing him to be lame. (If your horse does step on a nail, pull it out, clean the foot and bandage it until the veterinarian gets there. Ignore the myth that says no one but the vet should take the nail out. There's no reason why your horse should have to walk around with a nail in his foot until the veterinarian comes; that could increase the amount of damage done by the nail. Remember the place in the hoof from which you pulled the nail so that your veterinarian can explore the area.)

LOCATING THE LAMENESS

Although sometimes finding the location of a horse's lameness can be easy, at other times it can require a great deal of diagnostic skill and time. It may even take more than one examination to discover the source. Patience, on the part of the owner and the examiner, is a great asset to making an accurate diagnosis.

Not that people won't make you think that it's easy. All too frequently you will be watching your horse go around and someone will say, "Gee, I think he's moving a little stiff in the shoulder!" You will begin to wonder about your horse's shoulder and question whether or not you should have noticed something before. It's inevitable.

Horse people seem to think that all horse lameness, at least all front leg lameness, comes from the shoulder. If you want to impress your friends, don't say this. Shoulder lamenesses are extremely rare in the horse. The shoulder gets blamed for lameness because the horse does not want to reach forward to land on his foot when his leg is sore. The reason that he's not striding forward is usually not because of soreness in his shoulder but because he's trying to protect something in his leg. Usually it's his foot.

So, when you think you see a lame horse, if you have to impress your friends, say instead, "He's moving a little short—could be the foot." Since problems of the foot and its associated structures are the most common cause of lameness in the horse,[1] you will be right most of the time and you will impress your friends with your diagnostic skill. Forget the shoulder. Stop this myth.

Similarly, many people think that any time a horse "feels funny" in a hind leg the problem must be coming from the stifle area. Horses don't have nearly as many hind foot problems as they do forefoot problems, so the foot is not nearly as good a guess as to the source of a hind limb lameness as it is in the front limb. For that reason, if you are sitting on the fence and you insist on opining as to why the horse is lame, guess somewhere else. You probably hate it when your friends do this sort of thing to you, so guessing why *their* horse is lame from time to time is a good way to pay them back for your frustration.

Sometimes it's even hard to tell *whether* a horse is lame. If a horse is sore in both front feet, he may not know which leg to limp on, since both of them hurt. As such, he may appear to travel relatively sound.

The biggest myth of all about horse lameness is that you can ever tell if or when a particular horse is going to go lame. For example, X rays of the navicular bone cannot tell you if a horse is going to develop navicular disease. For that matter, X rays of *any* area are not that useful in telling what will be in the future for your horse.

The point is that when you talk about the "possibility" of a horse going lame, you are really just spinning your wheels. You might as well discuss the possibility of him getting run over by a truck if he lives near a road. Sure, things can happen. But no one knows enough to predict with any confidence whether or not they will.

Since it is not always possible to tell if a horse is lame or why it is lame and it is never possible to tell whether it is going to go lame, it should occur to you that lameness diagnosis is not a casual, offhand affair. As such, someone who looks at the way that a horse moves and says, "It looks like the stifle," is just being careless. Try to identify that your horse has a problem. Then call your veterinarian and take it from there.

"HEAD BOBBING" LAMENESS

How do you know if your horse is limping? The most obvious and most looked-for clinical sign of lameness is a bobbing head. That is, when the horse travels, his head, instead of being held steady, will bob up and down. The rhythmic bobbing, when it exists, gives the most obvious indication of where the lameness is. The horse's head and neck weigh three hundred pounds or so. That's a lot of weight to carry around. If one of the front legs is sore, the horse will try to avoid, to the extent that he can, having that weight hit the ground at the same time as his sore foot. Thus, he will lift his head up when the sore foot hits the ground. Or, alternatively, he will drop his head (and the extra weight) down onto the good foot. You can remember it either way: "Up on the bad foot" or "Down on the good foot"—just don't get them mixed up. The up-and-down movement of the head is most useful in the diagnosis of front leg lameness, but it is somewhat less useful when looking at hind legs or at problems involving multiple legs.

THE FLEXION TEST

Your veterinarian will employ a variety of diagnostic techniques to try and diagnose the cause of your horse's lameness (see Chapter One). One commonly employed test in evaluating lameness is the infamous flexion test.

For those of you familiar with lameness examinations and evaluations of horses that are being considered for purchase, flexion tests create myths, anxiety and confusion. During the flexion test, the examiner holds the front or back leg up in a flexed position for sixty or ninety seconds or so, depending on the leg and the examiner. The force with which the leg is flexed depends on who's doing it, too. Anyway, after a time, the horse is trotted off and he may or may not limp. He may limp so much you may think that he'll never trot sound again (since some horses can be quite dramatic), or he may "miss" a step or two upon trotting off. Or he may not limp at all.

If he doesn't limp, then you're home free because *not* limping after a flexion test is a result that cannot be misinterpreted. The flexed area will not be suspected as causing a problem for your horse. If he does limp, then you will have to deal with a lot of uncertainties as to the significance of that observation.

Normal horses can limp after flexion tests. Imagine that you've been asked to sit in a tight crouch for sixty seconds and then run right off. You might be a bit stiff. You might not be able to run at all. This might be because you have had knee problems in the past. You might be just fine but still be a bit stiff after this test.

In the same manner, flexion test examinations are useful, but not terribly accurate, screening tests for soreness in horse legs. In horses that are limping or that have chronic problems, a flexion test may increase pain and lameness. In horses with slight lameness, a flexion test may make a lameness easier to see and give the examiner a better indication of the general area in which a problem lies. But in and of themselves, and especially in horses that are clinically normal, flexion tests may not mean very much.

Flexion tests are certainly not very specific for the source of a problem. Each time that you flex a horse's leg, you bend a whole bunch of structures, from foot to knee in the front leg and from foot to hip in the hind. If your horse has a problem in *any* of these areas, he may limp following a flexion test.[2] And he may limp after this test even if he shows no signs of lameness otherwise.

The interpretation of flexion tests becomes particularly troubling during a routine prepurchase examination. Horse owners are occasionally flabbergasted by the fact that the horse that they are trying to sell, the one that has been sound for the last seven years, the one that has never refused a jump or missed a lead change, will sometimes hobble off after one of these flexion tests. Some purchasers (and their veterinarians) will use the results of these tests to decline purchase of an animal or to attempt to reduce the price. They will say that it "may" indicate an underlying problem. Of course, it may not. So if your horse doesn't "pass" a flexion test during a veterinary examination, don't panic (don't ever panic). He may just not like having his leg bent up. Or he may, in fact, have a problem that will need attention. But you almost never know whether or not there is a problem just by doing a flexion test.

Ideally, a flexion test will help your veterinarian find an answer to your horse's lameness problem so you can begin therapy. Let's hope the test won't be overinterpreted.

LIMB SWELLING

Having recognized that there is a problem in your horse's leg, you will want to treat it. Pain and swelling, when they exist, are generally signs of acute inflammation and should be treated.

Just because your horse has a swelling in his leg does not mean that there is something bad happening, by the way. Older horses frequently develop little swellings in and around their fetlock joints, for example, that you can't get rid of and that don't cause them any problems. These are called windpuffs (using the colorful vernacular of horse people of yore). A similar swelling in the hock is called a bog spavin. These swellings usually reflect that an area has received wear and tear over time.[3] Treating them is generally unnecessary and unrewarding since they almost never bother the horse and you generally can't make them go away. No one really knows what causes them in the first place. (The medical community refers to this sort of condition as idiopathic, meaning nobody knows just exactly what's going on.) Just consider these unsightly bulges jewelry for your horse, that is, something that he's going to enjoy wearing for a long time.

One of the great things about the way that horses are put together is that if you are not sure if something is normal, there are three other legs that look just the same as the one you are worried about (in the lower parts, anyway). If the swelling looks the same on one leg as it does on another, chances are that the "problem" is just a variation of normal for your horse, rather than a simultaneous occurrence of abnormality in both legs.

When a swelling occurs because of inflammation, it almost always is associated with pain and heat in the affected area and in most cases lameness. If a swelling isn't painful to the touch (make sure your horse isn't just irritated by the fact that you are touching him), or isn't painful when you manipulate the area, or he isn't limping, or if an identical swelling exists on another leg, it's probably insignificant. If there is a painful area on the leg that is swollen, it's probably best to call your veterinarian to get some advice on how to take care of it.

BANDAGING

Bandaging an injured leg is a good way to help control swelling and inflammation. Bandaging reduces movement, which helps to control pain, too. Bandages also provide some support for the healing tissues.[4] Leg bandages are also frequently used in athletic horses. They are supposed to provide protection from trauma, to support the bandaged legs and to absorb some of the energy transmitted to the legs as the horse moves. Do they?

Surprisingly few studies have been done on the use of bandages in athletic horses. That bandages should provide protection to the legs seems evident, and no one is going bother studying that. But there have been very few studies on the support and energy absorption provided by bandages.

A leg is "supported" to try to keep it from stretching or bending too much at the level of the fetlock joint. Support means that the wrap will attempt to resist the cannon bone's tendency to go down into the ground when the fetlock joint bends as the horse travels forward. When a horse moves, the fetlock joint, which flexes back when the leg is in the air, flexes the other way (dorsiflexes) when the leg hits the ground. As a result, all of the tendons and ligaments on the back side of the leg stretch. With a support wrap, you are trying to resist this stretching.

Support to a leg can be provided by a bandage. For it to work, however, a wrap must go down below the fetlock and around the pastern. According to the research, the tighter the wrap, the more support you get. The support from a tight wrap wears off more quickly than that provided by a moderately tight wrap, however. A bandage that goes only around the cannon bone probably does not provide any significant support, although it does provide some protection from external trauma (and a colorful counterpoint to your horse's natural color). Support wraps evidently also absorb some of the energy received by the leg, although the amount of energy absorption varies depending on the type of material used and the way that the bandage is applied.[5,6]

Unfortunately, all wraps loosen fairly quickly as the leg bends repeatedly (within minutes), and the amount of true support that you get from a bandage decreases rapidly and accordingly. Nonetheless, many performance horses are wrapped for support. Support wraps are certainly a good idea unless they are applied *too* tightly (remember, the *direction* doesn't matter!).

There are many types of boots available to provide support to legs, too. Unfortunately, their effectiveness is questionable, and to date no one has published any good research on them. The boots certainly look good; heck, many of them look just like they have come from the very cutting edge of advanced equine technology. Boots, too, provide some external protection to the leg (as well as color). But who knows how well they work to provide support?

If you want to wrap your horse's legs for support, go ahead. Use boots instead if you want. But after a few minutes of the horse jogging around and loosening things up, how much support he *actually* gets from wraps is yet to be determined. A properly applied support wrap probably does *some* good.

You can bandage your horse's legs, or not, to control the swelling that many horses get from standing around in a stall. This is commonly referred to as stocking up. Stocking up can occur in some horses solely because of inactivity. Exercise has an important mechanical pumping effect that helps remove fluid from the horse's legs. Several days without exercise (or even overnight) can cause some horses' legs to swell up. Stocking up in a limb can also occur as a result of scar tissue from a previous infection or injury.

This type of swelling will usually disappear rapidly with exercise and the leg will look normal within minutes. When you come back the next day, the leg may be swollen all over again, but it will not be painful and the horse will never limp. If you don't like the way the leg looks when it's swollen, keep it wrapped. If it doesn't bother you or your horse, you can generally let the leg swell. If your horse is in a situation where he can walk around and pump his leg up and down regularly, like a pasture instead of a box stall, the swelling will most likely take care of itself.

There's a myth that if a horse is kept wrapped all the time, it will become "dependent" on the wraps. What does this mean? What will they depend on? If the legs swell without wraps, then wraps will help control the swelling. If the legs don't swell, wrapping then won't make them start, unless you injure them by wrapping as tightly as you can. A leg won't get "weaker" because it is wrapped.

LAMENESS AND CONFORMATION

You cannot predict lameness by recognizing that a horse's conformation is "undesirable." Conformation is the way the horse is supposed to be put together, as opposed to the way that he is put together. Those who devote time and energy to the study of horse conformation assert that certain conformational abnormalities will predispose a horse to leg and lameness problems.

Much of conformation analysis is devoted to deciding in what way the horse's leg deviates from the ideal line, and it's sort of like judging a beauty pageant. The horse leg resembles a cylinder that drops down from the shoulder or flank. If there is deviation from the ideal way this cylinder is formed, the story goes, extra stress will be put on certain parts of the horse's leg as he moves, "predisposing" the horse to problems in the stressed areas.[7]

When a horse strides, all his weight comes over the top of the leg. Theoretically, anyway, if all of the parts line up just right, then the stress will be distributed as evenly as possible over the whole limb. Since stress is always delivered at a ninety-degree angle to the ground (due to the force of gravity), areas of the leg that are out of line will theoretically receive extra stress and be more prone to injury than the parts that are within the line. For example, if the horse is back at the knee, then theoretically there will be more stress on the front of the knee when the horse strides over the leg. This may "predispose" him to chip fractures. Similarly, conversations about predisposition to things like splints (that occur along the cannon bone) and tendon injuries occur.

To use a different species as an example, look at dogs. It probably comes as no surprise to you that Dachshunds have back problems or that English Bulldogs have breathing problems. Look at them! But not all Dachshunds and Bulldogs have these problems. If you are considering buying one of these dogs, do you decide against doing so because of its potential problems? The situation in horses is analogous.

Whether conformational "abnormalities" actually mean anything is anyone's guess. So far, no one has ever done a study evaluating the conformation of a group of horses and then observing the horses for several years to see if problems develop in those horses with "poor" conformation. Such a study would be tremendously interesting and useful, but it would be very hard to observe a number of individual horses for the several years that would be required to complete it.

The point is, if you like a horse, you shouldn't necessarily be dissuaded from purchasing him just because his conformation is not the way it's supposed to be. Virtually no horse has ideal conformation. Even with extreme variations in conformation, low-level exercise, like trail riding, may not be enough of a stress to cause problems anyway.[8]

This is not to say that conformational analysis is without benefit. For instance, it is well known that if a horse stands with his toes turned way out, it will cause his hooves to swing to the inside as he travels forward. You can predict that he may whack himself on the ankles as he travels forward. Such trauma can cause cuts, swelling and soreness. But not all horses that toe out will hit their ankles.

Be careful not to overinterpret a horse. If the book says that your horse's legs aren't straight enough and the book says that this may predispose him to lameness and the book says that since he's off after a flexion test his joints must hurt and the book says that he's not supposed to have a swelling where one exists, then sit back and remember one thing. He may be just fine. Horses don't read books.

ARTHRITIS

Horses tend to get arthritic conditions, both acute and chronic, and much diagnostic and therapeutic effort goes into the treatment and control of them.

Horse people like to have names for things. If a veterinarian says, "The horse has degenerative arthritis of the distal intertarsal joint," the client will walk away shaking his or her head and wondering what in the world the vet was talking about and why he or she insists on using those big words. But if the vet says, "The horse has bone spavin," the client is generally very happy that at least the condition can be called something.

There are names for all sorts of conditions of horses that date back to the 1700s and earlier. Horse people still use them, and although the names are a colorful and quaint part of equine medicine, they are not particularly useful, except as buzz words that can be used around the barn. The names, however, tend to obscure what is really going on. Nevertheless, you have "bog spavin" and "bone spavin" and "blood spavin" and "jack spavin" and "ringbone" and a whole bunch of other great-sounding names that were dreamed up to give a name to arthritic conditions of the horse. It will do you good to get beyond the names so you can begin to understand your horse's real problems.

What is arthritis anyway? Arthritis occurs in a joint. A joint occurs anywhere that two bones meet. The ends of the bones in a joint are covered with cartilage, a smooth tissue that allows the ends of the bones to glide over the top of each other with a minimum of friction. Within the joint is the joint fluid (synovial fluid). This fluid has two primary functions: to supply nourishment to the cartilage and to lubricate the joint. The joint capsule is made up of all the tissue surrounding the joint.

Arthritis is, by definition, inflammation of a joint. It may be either acute or chronic.

ACUTE VS. CHRONIC ARTHRITIS

Acute arthritis is that which comes up immediately, like a sprained ankle in a person. Acute arthritis can get better. The cause of acute arthritis is generally related to some form of injury. Importantly, *not all horses that have an episode of acute arthritis will develop chronic arthritis* (although acute inflammation of a joint can start a horse down the path to chronic arthritis).

Chronic (degenerative) arthritis, like any form of chronic inflammation, is a long-term process. You can never get rid of it, and it will most likely get worse with time (hence the term "degenerative"). No one knows why chronic arthritis develops in a particular animal.

The signs of acute inflammation may actually decrease if the situation becomes chronic. If your horse has acute arthritis, you may feel that the area is hot or swollen and you may see that your horse is limping. If your horse has chronic arthritis, you will generally not find much heat and sometimes there will be little swelling. Pain, however, will be a feature of both diseases. It is what happens inside the chronically inflamed joint that makes this condition so interesting to veterinarians, but at the same time so frustrating and difficult to treat.

HOW ARTHRITIS DEVELOPS

Cartilage is bound to the bone like white on rice. When a joint becomes inflamed, byproducts of inflammation are released into the joint. These byproducts are very destructive to cartilage and they begin to degrade it. Cartilage does attempt to repair itself, but the repair process that cartilage undergoes is almost never effective at healing the injured tissue (cartilage healing is an area of ongoing research).[9] Therefore, over time, the layer of cartilage that protects the bone will begin to wear out.

As an arthritic condition develops, the extent of the wearing down of the cartilage cannot be adequately evaluated without directly looking at it (with an arthroscope, for instance). Cartilage is mostly water and does not show up on X rays. Therefore, X rays will not tell you if there is minor cartilage damage in an arthritic joint, that is, cartilage damage that has occurred without damage to the underlying bone. That's part of the reason why arthritis can be so insidious; it can go unrecognized.

As cartilage damage continues and arthritis becomes chronic, the underlying bone is revealed. This causes inflammation in the bone of the joint. Bone resents being inflamed. Bone responds to inflammation by becoming active and creating more bone. (This is one of the reasons why your arm heals after you break it.) When bone begins to be produced in a joint, there are no longer smooth, gliding surfaces to rub up against each other. Rather, there are rough, bony surfaces. As the bone continues to grind and more bone is produced, characteristic changes begin to show up in the horse. The horse gets lame, for example. The joint may become very painful, especially to a flexion test (the tests can be useful). Changes from the normal X-ray appearance of the joint may begin to show up as the joint continues to deteriorate. Bone "spurring" and "lipping" are early X-ray signs that indicate that things are going downhill in the joint. Once these changes have occurred, the condition is, unfortunately, irreversible.[9] No one can return a degenerating joint to normal.

The formation of new bone in an arthritic joint gives rise to the colorful names that are used to identify arthritis in the horse. "Ringbone" refers to the ring of bone that forms around one of the two joints of the horse's pastern as the joint deteriorates. Horse people sometimes wonder why you cannot cure ringbone by chipping away the ring of bone. The ring of bone isn't the problem. The fact that there is not much good cartilage left in the joint is.

"Spavin" refers to the same process of cartilage degeneration in the lower joints of the hock. This is a very old term, and the meaning is obscure. The term is quite versatile, however. "Bog spavin" describes a swollen tibiotarsal joint (the joint in which most of the hock motion occurs), and "bone spavin" is used to describe arthritis of the lower joints of the hock. Terms like "blind spavin" and "jack spavin" and "blood spavin" are not at all specific, however, and they can be apparently used with impunity to describe any particular condition the describer wishes to name. Isn't it easier just to call the stuff arthritis?

TREATMENT

When a horse has arthritis, he may be treated with one of a variety of products that try to help relieve pain and inflammation, restore the environment of the joint to normal, control swelling or otherwise fight off the problem. These products may be given systemically (in the horse's system, orally or by injection) or by injection into the joint.

Acute cases of arthritis can subside with no permanent or long-lasting effects. With chronic arthritis, treatment involves trying to help the horse handle his soreness by making his life as pain-free as possible. Paradoxically, in some cases of chronic arthritis, when things get really bad, the horse will be just fine!

A few joints in the horse's body really don't seem to serve much purpose. The pastern joint and the lowest two hock joints are cases in point. These joints don't move very much at all. It is possible for the deterioration in the joints to reach such an advanced stage—to have so much new bone production as a result of the arthritic process—that the two sides of the joint just grow together. When this happens, the joint is, for all practical purposes, fused into one solid bone and there is no more motion in the joint, no more bone grinding on bone. As a result the horse can go completely sound. This can occur "naturally" in some horses. Joint fusion can be hastened by local injection or surgery in some cases, too.[10,11,12]

Unfortunately, in many cases arthritis does have career-ending consequences. For these horses, light exercise and regular administration of anti-inflammatory pain-relieving drugs like phenylbutazone is the best help that veterinarians can offer. Some horses just can't be helped much at all.

Not that other help isn't offered from other sources. Once a diagnosis of degenerative arthritis has been secured, there will be all sorts of products and advice for you to choose from. A mountain of supplements and anti-inflammatory "natural" products are available. You may hear from an acupuncturist. You may look into lasers or magnets or ultrasound or any number of nonproven, generally ineffective treatments. At least, to save yourself a lot of disappointment, don't expect much help from these sorts of things because the joint just can't be returned to normal. Don't give up trying to help your horse and don't give up hope that he can be helped, but also be realistic if you are faced with the often difficult problem of chronic degenerative arthritis.

TENDON INJURIES

A tendon connects a muscle to bone. When a muscle contracts (the only thing that muscle can do), it pulls on the bone via the tendon. These are important structures.

There are two large and very important tendons that run down the back of the horse's leg. The superficial flexor tendon is, as the name implies, closest to the surface. Immediately underneath it lies the deep flexor tendon. For performance horses, injury to either of these structures can mean trouble. As a final bit of tendon anatomy, you will hear about the tendon sheath. A sheath lets a tendon glide through a turn around the back of a joint, as occurs behind the fetlock or knee (carpus) of the horse. The tendon sheath is a fluid-filled cover for the tendon. This structure can get injured, too. A lot of people think that a tendon sheath runs all the way up the lower leg, but it doesn't; the two sheaths of the lower leg cover only about the upper and lower thirds of the back of the lower leg.

Tendons are normally a little bit elastic. When the leg hits the ground, the tendons will stretch just a bit before pulling the leg back up off the ground as the muscles of the back of the leg contract. This is thought to help relieve some of the stress on the leg.

Tendons are constructed something like a cable. That is, they are one big fiber composed of a lot of little fibers running together. Tendons are quite resilient under normal circumstances, but like anything else, if they get overused bad things can happen.

When horses are asked to do things that they normally wouldn't do (if given a choice), like jump bunches of fences in a row or run really fast and far until they are almost exhausted, a potential for injury to the tendons exists. Each time that the tendons and muscles stretch and contract, they get tired. As they fatigue, they lose their normal springiness. Tired tendons begin to stretch and *not* recoil.

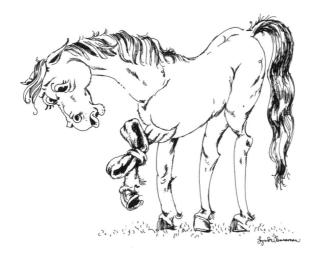

Watch out for a bowed tendon!

This whole affair is sort of like what happens when you bend a paper clip back and forth. The paper clip can take a good bit of bending, but each time that you bend it back and forth, a little bit of metal gives. The paper clip very rapidly becomes easy to bend until it breaks.

Apparently, most tendon injuries occur in this way. That is, a tendon is repeatedly overstressed until finally something gives. In some cases, tendon injuries may occur due to a single instance of overload, but this is evidently much less common than injuries caused by repeated stress. When a tendon gives, you will then be confronted with the dreaded "bowed" tendon.

SIGNS OF AN INJURED TENDON

The name "bowed" tendon refers to the characteristic appearance of an injured tendon. Instead of the normal flat appearance at the back of the lower leg, the tendon will swell out, giving the leg a bow-shaped appearance.

Besides swelling, the other classic signs of inflammation also occur when a tendon is injured. The swelling will be painful, especially if it is pinched when the leg is off the ground. The area may be hot. The horse will generally limp, reflecting a loss of function, unless the injury is quite mild.

TREATMENT OF AN INJURED TENDON

When a tendon injury is suspected, three things must be done so that the best healing can be achieved. First, the acute inflammation must be controlled.

Second, the extent of the injury must be recognized. Third, the injury must be given time to heal.

As with any acutely inflamed area, treatment of the acutely injured tendon is designed to control all of the signs of inflammation. Especially important is controlling the swelling. Swelling is really bad for a tendon. Swelling takes up space in the tendon. The more a tendon is allowed to swell, the more the fibers in the tendon are disrupted and displaced and the more tendon damage occurs. Local application of cold therapy, bandaging and anti-inflammatory drugs are used to control the swelling. In addition, the horse should be strictly confined to prevent further tendon damage, which can be incurred if the tissue is further stressed by excess motion.[13,14]

The second important thing to do is to recognize the extent of the injury. A swollen, sore and hot tendon is usually pretty obvious. But not all hot, swollen and sore tendons are badly injured. Proper treatment requires knowing exactly what is injured and how badly it is hurt.

This recognition involves the use of diagnostic ultrasound. By now, everyone in veterinary medicine should have figured out that it is impossible to diagnose accurately what is going on inside a horse's injured tendon without the use of an ultrasound machine. (In addition to the two tendons, there are two other major supporting structures in the lower leg of the horse, the suspensory ligament and the inferior check ligament, and while these structures are different in form and function from the tendons, they are injured in much the same way.) It is not possible to determine the extent of an injury to these structures without ultrasound, nor is it always possible to determine which structure is injured without the use of this technique. Sometimes, relatively minor swellings conceal a relatively extensive injury. Sometimes legs that are remarkably swollen, sore and hot have no underlying tendon damage. If diagnostic ultrasound is available to you when your horse hurts a tendon, you really should take advantage of the opportunity to find out exactly what's wrong.[15]

Finally, the third important thing to realize about tendon injuries is that they take time to heal—a lot of time. Tendons, due to the nature of the tissue, are unable to repair themselves with normal tendon. Instead, the tendon tissue is replaced with scar tissue. Scar tissue, unfortunately, is not as strong as normal tendon. It's strong enough, in most cases anyway, so that the horse can eventually return to work. Newly formed scar tissue takes time to strengthen and mature, however. It may take as long as a year, in the case of a serious injury, for the tendon to regain its ultimate strength.

Patience, then, is an invaluable asset in dealing with tendon injuries. Since patience is not a commodity that is in great supply with many horse owners, however, there is a natural and unfortunate tendency to try to speed up the healing process. So far, *nothing* has been discovered or invented that will speed up tendon healing. Remember that the next time someone tries to sell you something.

In the treatment of an injured tendon, occasionally surgery may be recommended. In certain tendon injuries, those that have occurred with a large tear in the center of the tissue, creating a core of injured tissue (like a jelly doughnut, where the jelly is the injury), it has been shown that letting the fluid out of the core is beneficial in promoting healing. This is done by stabbing the tendon (under local anesthesia, of course) with a scalpel blade. By relieving the fluid buildup, the tendon tissue can reduce in size and then begin to try to repair itself.

Tendon surgery is neither necessary nor suitable for all tendon injuries. It is useful in the core lesions described above but not very useful in other types of tears. The healing that tendon surgery promotes has nothing to do with bringing "increased circulation" into the tendon, as veterinarians used to believe when the technique was first described years ago. The surgery merely helps release the fluid in the core of the tendon, sort of like popping a blister on your finger.[16]

Another type of surgery may be recommended for injuries of the superficial flexor tendon only. Behind the horse's knee (carpus) is a structure known as the superior check ligament (not to be confused with the inferior check ligament, lower in the leg). The superior check ligament is thought to help resist the downward pull on the superficial flexor tendon that occurs when a horse bears weight. That is, when the horse steps and puts weight on his leg, the stretching of the superficial tendon is apparently "checked" by this ligament.

In the treatment of some superficial flexor tendon injuries, surgical transection (cutting) of the superior check ligament may be advised, so that the tendon can stretch a bit more when the horse bears weight and, it is hoped, be less likely to tear further.[17]

It is important to note that veterinarians are carefully studying both types of surgeries for tendon injury. The popularity of these surgeries comes and goes as new studies are released. As with most of medicine, there are rarely "right" answers, only options.

Tendon injuries do take time to heal, but it has been well demonstrated that time alone does not promote the most effective healing. The healing of a tendon injury should occur under some sort of stress. That is, the healing that occurs in the tendon can be helped by the application of *mild* exercise stress to the leg. In the horse, this means that early in the post-injury recovery period, the horse should begin walking. This early exercise will encourage the healing to occur in a coordinated fashion, resulting in healing tissue that is laid down along the lines of stress, in the way that it will be the strongest.[14] Of course, you don't want to go too fast; you could run the risk of reinjury if you do that. That's why follow-up examinations are in order as your horse's tendon heals after injury.

Ultimately, for most performance horses, tendon injuries have a good end result, and the horse can usually return to full work, albeit with a bit of an enlarged leg. In racing horses, however, an injured tendon, even if it is fully repaired, may not be strong enough to withstand the rigors of high-speed work. Tendon injuries have spelled the end of the road for many a racehorse. But for most horses, given time and proper treatment, rest and rehabilitation, the tendon will get better. The time will pass slowly, but it will pass.

When you are trying to find out information about horse legs, the best way to avoid undue frustration for yourself is to limit your sources of information. You or your horse trainer should decide if the horse isn't moving right. Let your horseshoer put shoes on his feet. Let your veterinarian give you information as to what is wrong with his leg. If you want another opinion, go to another veterinarian. Ask questions and gather information from *informed* sources. Smile at your friends when they tell you what to do. Don't listen too closely and thank them sincerely for their help (you will want to keep them as friends). Then go on and take care of your horse's legs reasonably and rationally.

14

Hooves

"No foot, no horse." This much horse people know. And they know a lot of myths, too.

People are terribly bothered by the fact that experts don't know everything. Not enough research has been done to explain some things. Other things defy explanation and are just unknowable. Since it's not possible to know everything, most people just make up the answers as they go along. They become experts about talking about how things *should* be. They often ignore the way things are. If you are fortunate enough to find experts who can admit to you that they don't know everything, hold on to them tightly. At least they are telling you the truth.

Veterinarians and farriers can look at a horse's foot and think about what should be, particularly with regard to horseshoeing and "proper" hoof care. In most cases, unfortunately, no one really *knows* what the results of changing things about a horse's hooves will be.

Surprisingly little research has been done on how shoeing affects the horse's leg. Much of traditional horseshoeing theory is based on principles that are literally hundreds of years old. That's not to say that the theories are incorrect; it does, however, suggest that principles that are this old must be long cherished and difficult to challenge.

But some scientific studies have been done on the effects of shoeing and trimming on the movement of the leg. What appears in the studies is contrary to many things people think should happen. This presents a dilemma. The occurrence of contradictory facts may require a change of mind. If the facts get in the way of what people think *should* happen, they tend to just ignore the facts.

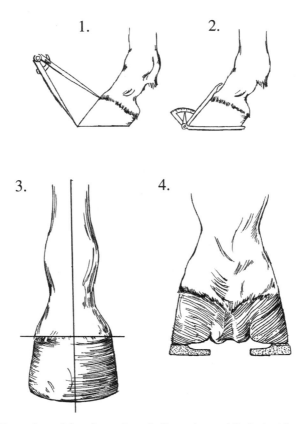

The hoof is evaluated for: 1. toe length; 2. angle; and 3. & 4. side-to-side balance.

The foot is the center of a lot of activity in the horse. All of the horse's weight lands on the foot. The majority of the lameness problems in the horse can be attributed to the front feet.[1,2] The feet, especially the front feet, are obviously a very important area.

THE SHAPE OF THE HOOF

First, you need to understand some basic terminology to help you look at the feet. If the bottom of the foot is level with the ground, the front of the hoof wall forms an angle with the ground (and the bottom of the foot). The angle of the front foot in most horses is from 50 to 55 degrees. The angle of the hind foot is generally slightly steeper, between 53 and 57 degrees.[2,3,4] Some people and some texts will tell you that "normal" horse hoof angles are lower than this. No, they are not.

Horses can vary within these ranges and be normal. If the hoof angle is too steep, that is, the heel is too long or the toe is too short, the horse may have what is commonly called a club foot. If the angle is too shallow, that is, the heel is too short or the toe is too long, the heel is said to be underslung. The hoof angle is easy to change by raising or lowering the heel or toe.

The proper angle of the foot is said by some to be the same as the angle of the shoulder. This is determined by a line from the crest of the withers and through the point of the shoulder that intersects with the line of the ground.[5] As you might imagine, this is not the easiest measure to obtain with repeatability and precision (two things that you should demand of *any* measurement), since it's sometimes difficult to figure out exactly where these points are on a particular horse (say, a fat horse or one with no clearly defined withers).

Therefore, another, more commonly used way to determine the proper angle for an individual horse is by trying to ensure that there is a continuous line from the fetlock to the ground. That is, the angle that the hoof wall forms with the ground should extend all the way to the fetlock joint in a straight line.[4,6]

If the heel is very high or very short and underslung, the horse is said to have a broken hoof/pastern axis. This is very bad, according to some, and it is not desirable in the author's experience, either. However, the bad things that might happen in the *future* as a result of a broken axis have never actually been demonstrated. No one has ever taken a group of horses, identified that they have this problem, left the problem alone (and not tried to fix it) and then followed the horses to see what happens to them.

The "balance" of the foot refers to the length of the sides of the feet in comparison to each other. A balanced foot is the same length on each side of the hoof wall.[3]

Finally, the length of the foot is pretty important. If a horse's foot is too short, there may not be enough foot underneath the bone to protect it from concussion and bruising when the foot hits the ground. A horse with too short a foot gets very sore very quickly. Conversely, a horse with too long a foot may stumble or move awkwardly.

Nearly everyone measures the length of the foot from the coronary band to the ground, down the front of the toe. It's been done this way since the time of Alexander the Great. (Apparently, no one has found a better way to measure the length of the foot in the interim.) Anyway, there are some useful guidelines that you can follow as to how long your horse's foot should be after it is trimmed. For small horses, say 800 to 900 pounds, the toe length could be 3 inches. For medium-size horses, 950 to 1,050 pounds, the toe length could be trimmed to $3^1/_4$ inches. For big horses, over 1,150 pounds, a toe length of $3^1/_2$ inches is appropriate.[3]

These are general guidelines, not hard-and-fast rules.

When looking for hoof problems in your horse, keep these three things in mind: (1) the foot should be level and balanced from side to side; (2) the foot should be at an angle that is within the normal range and also appears normal for that horse; and (3) the foot should be at an appropriate length for the size of the horse. If these three things are consistently accomplished, you will go a long way toward keeping your horse traveling sound.

THE "FLIGHT" OF THE HOOF

When the horse strides, the hoof is on the ground for a while; then it is picked up and carried through the air. When the hoof is in the air, not much interesting happens to it (although the foot does not trace an arc through the air, as most people think).[7] People who attempt to manipulate the foot concern themselves with what happens when the horse's hoof is landing on the ground.

There have been very few studies looking at how the horse's foot normally lands on the ground. Naturally, *some* part of the hoof hits the ground first. At the trot, in some of the horses studied, the heel hits first. In most horses, the foot lands flat. In none of the normal trotting horses examined does the toe land first.[7,8] But there is variation among how horses' feet normally land.

Not only is there no right way for the hoof to land, but it has been shown that the foot lands differently at different gaits.[9] If you or your farrier are absolutely adamant that your horse must land flat, you have to realize that you may be in for some frustration trying to make it so at all gaits. Seeing that the horse's foot lands flat at the walk by no means assures you that it will land the same way at the trot and canter. Furthermore, this begs the question of whether or not landing flat is that important anyway, since many normal horses land heel first. Finally, even if you could establish that the horse was landing flat on level ground, it still might not help much if the horse travels over uneven terrain, such as occurs in most plowed show rings, trails or, for that matter, anywhere else that isn't paved. On these surfaces, landing flat is probably impossible.

What does seem to be consistent is that no matter how the hoof lands on the ground, the inside of the foot takes the hardest pounding. This makes some sense, since the inside of the foot is the part most underneath the horse's body. In fact, you can radically change the way that a horse's foot is balanced from side to side or front to back and he will still land with most of his weight on the inside of his foot. In one study, the side-to-side balance was altered by about $^3/_4$ inch (about $^3/_8$ inch in either direction) and although weight distribution changed with balance, the inside of the foot always hit hardest.[9] What this suggests is that a lot of the changes that are made to alter the hoof balance of a horse by $^1/_{16}$ inch here or there may not make all that much difference in the stress that is applied to the foot as the horse travels.

BREAKOVER

"Breakover" is another buzz word that refers to how the foot leaves the ground. A horse must rotate his foot over his toe (break over) as his foot comes off the ground when the leg goes forward.

All sorts of manipulations are done to change the speed with which a horse breaks over his toe. It makes sense that if you roll the toe of the hoof or shoe, if you curve the toe up, the foot will roll over the front of the toe and his breakover will be faster and easier, right? Similarly, if you were to raise the heel (and pitch the horse forward on his foot), you might think you could speed up the breakover as well (since the horse would be theoretically closer to falling over the front of the foot anyway).

There are all sorts of reasons why you might want to increase breakover. For instance, if your horse had some stiffness from arthritis of the lower leg, wouldn't it be nice if you could help him roll over his toe just a little easier? Or if your horse tended to step on his front heels with his hind foot, wouldn't it be nice if you could get the front foot out of the way a little quicker by speeding breakover?

High-speed, slow-motion photography shows that breakover can be affected by shoeing. Generally, if you lengthen the horse's toe, you will slow down his breakover at the trot.[7,8,9] But the change in breakover doesn't appear to be consistent at all gaits; that is, just because his breakover is slower at the walk doesn't mean that it will be slower at the trot and canter as well.[9] Similarly, if you elevate a horse's heel, the speed of the breakover can be increased slightly, though inconsistently.

What's really curious is that just about *any* alteration on the foot will change the breakover. Breakover is changed by application of thick and thin pads under the shoe. It's also affected if you elevate the inside or outside part of the foot. None of the alterations affect all horses the same way at all gaits.[9] As a practical matter, nobody can realistically predict what *any* shoeing change is going to do to a particular horse's breakover. However, just about any shoeing change is going to do *something*.

TOE LENGTH VS. STRIDE LENGTH

It has long been said that if you lengthen the horse's toe, you will lengthen the horse's stride. Racehorses, in particular, are trimmed so that their toes are really long and their heels are really short. This long toe is supposed to make it more difficult for the horse to break over. The idea is that if the foot takes longer to break over, the horse will have to pick his foot up higher when he strides. If he picks his foot up high, the myth goes, then he will reach out more and cover more ground with each stride. Longer stride, faster horse, right?

Wrong. Photography shows that a long toe doesn't make a bit of difference in the length of the stride. It does alter slightly the path that the foot takes through the air, but it does not change the distance covered by each stride.[7,8,9] The only thing that you do by lengthening the toe or lowering the heel is make the horse tend to land either flat or on his toe.[7,8] Some horses will still land on their heel first if the toe is lengthened, but more of them will land flat or *toe* first than if the foot is kept at a normal angle. Normal horses generally don't land on their toes first.

It's amazing how something like this long toe/long stride myth persists. It persists in spite of data that show that more horses with lameness related to the hoof tend to have a long toe/low heel conformation than do horses with normal hoof angles.[2] It persists in spite of data that show that problems that prevent racing or training are significantly higher in horses with long toe/low heel conformation than in horses with normal angles.[10]

Changing horse hoof angles is relatively easy. Changing peoples' minds is relatively impossible.

HEEL ELEVATION AND HOOF ANGLE CHANGES

Heel elevation is prescribed sometimes as a treatment for tendon injuries, to take the pressure off the tendon. It doesn't work. Two studies have measured the strain in the major tendons and ligaments of the foreleg and how it changes when the horse's foot was adjusted from 40 degrees (lower than you've ever seen) to 70 degrees (higher than you've ever thought possible) and from 55 to 78 degrees. With heel elevation, there is no change in the strain of the superficial flexor tendon.[11,12] There *is* a slight decrease in the strain on the deep flexor tendon as the angle is made steeper, but the hoof angle must change by *fifteen degrees* to see anything significant.[11] (This actually makes some sense, since the deep flexor tendon is the only one of these important structures that goes all the way down to the foot.) The point is, if you have tendon problems, don't expect angle changes in the foot to do any good in treating or preventing problems for your horse.

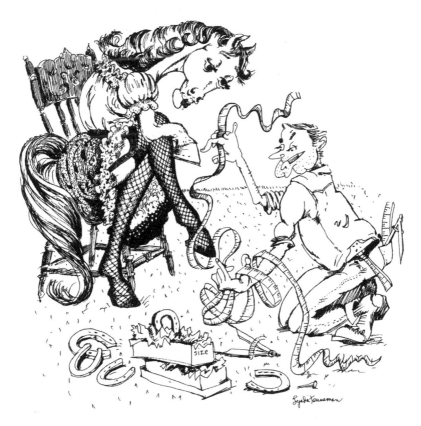

Proper shoeing involves careful attention to the foot.

At best, raising the horse's heel does nothing to alleviate strain in the suspensory ligament.[11,12] If your horse has a suspensory ligament injury, however, raising the heel may even be harmful. With heel elevation, one study showed an increase in suspensory ligament strain,[13] while another showed an *increase* in the strain of the lower branches of the ligament.[12] This would almost certainly be harmful in a horse that is trying to recover from an injury to this area.

Elevating a horse's heel is often done with a wedge pad under the heel. Even this apparently innocuous change has significant effects on the hoof. Adding heel wedges increases strain in the hoof wall in the quarters and actually *decreases* strain in the toe, which is exactly the opposite of what most people think.[12]

Shoeing-angle changes don't affect the bones of the lower leg in the ways that most people think, either. Shoeing-angle changes are sometimes prescribed to help relieve the pressure on arthritic or degenerative bones, especially in the treatment of arthritis of the pastern (ringbone) or in therapy for navicular disease.

Hoof-angle changes affect the fetlock joint very little. An increase in the hoof angle causes a *decrease* in the angle of the fetlock joint. But to get a one degree change in the fetlock joint, you have to alter the hoof angle by *ten* degrees.[14] For all practical purposes, this isn't possible in a horse in which normal movement is desired.

Other joints are affected slightly more by shoeing-angle changes than is the fetlock. To move the pastern joint by one degree, the hoof angle has to be changed by three degrees.[14] The coffin joint is very much affected by hoof-angle changes. The orientation of the coffin joint is affected on an almost 1:1 basis by hoof-angle changes; that is, each degree in hoof-angle change affects the coffin-joint angle by almost the same amount.[12,14]

THE EFFECT OF SHOEING CHANGES

What does all this mean for your horse?

Good question.

Basically, it means that if you change your horse's hoof angle and toe length and foot balance you are likely to do something to your horse's lower leg. You may not be able to predict how the changes you make will affect the movement of the leg. In many cases the changes you actually get may be completely different from what you have heard or think will happen. Even though there are a few studies showing what happens to the foot as a result of shoeing changes, there are almost none showing how lame horses respond to them.

You may well ask in frustration, "Why shoe the darn thing anyway if no one knows if it's going to make any difference?"

The primary reason to shoe a horse is to keep his foot from wearing out. The shoe protects the foot. Ground is to hoof what sandpaper is to wood. You *need* to shoe your horse if you ride him a lot on abrasive ground. If he's in a soft pasture or if he has very hard feet or if he isn't ridden very often, he probably doesn't need shoes at all.

"What about all these therapeutic shoes?" you ask.

Let's put things in perspective: This chapter is not trying to say that shoeing a horse isn't important. Nor is it trying to say that shoeing changes can't help (or hinder) your horse. Many horses travel better because they are shod, and therapeutic shoes can be very helpful in treating certain conditions. Bar shoes, for example, a type of shoe with a metal bar across the back, in one of a variety of configurations, can sometimes be very useful in the treatment of conditions associated with heel soreness.[15] However, bar shoes can make some horses sore in the heels, too.

Shoeing a horse can be something of a double-edged sword. Even though shoes are very useful in protecting the feet, they may also tend to inhibit the natural action of the foot in absorbing shock. When the hoof lands on the ground, it expands. Hoof expansion acts as a shock absorber.[16] You can demonstrate the same sort of action by placing your hand on a countertop. If you cup your hand slightly, you can hit the back of your cupped hand with your other fist surprisingly hard without causing pain. This is because the expansion of your hand helps distribute pressure. In a similar fashion, the foot expands and relieves some of the stress when the leg hits the ground.

Horseshoes are rigid objects. It seems reasonable to think that they could inhibit the expansion of the foot. And because they are also nailed to the hoof wall, they could also tend to concentrate stress in this area. Thus, it would follow that a horseshoe, especially if poorly applied, could *hurt* your horse by preventing normal foot expansion and increasing stress to certain areas of the foot.

The point is this: Shoeing a horse is as much of an art as it is a science. It may be impossible to predict what will actually happen to a horse when his feet are trimmed and when shoes are nailed onto his feet. There are a tremendous number of theories about shoeing and hoof balance, and a good farrier or a good veterinarian should be familiar with many of them. Ideally, one of those theories will end up helping your horse if he has a problem in his hoof.

Give your farrier and your veterinarian a break. If your horse has a problem with his foot, they have to look at it and, based on their experience, try to figure out what might be the best way to help that particular problem. Experience, though, is just the end product of a bunch of mistakes. Let them try things on your horse's foot, and if they don't work out the first time, give the people another shot at the problem. Unfortunately, just because they think something should work a certain way doesn't mean that it will.

SOLVING HOOF PROBLEMS

Myth #1 about treating feet, as told by veterinarians: "Farriers don't know anything about horse feet."

Myth #2 about treating feet, as told by farriers: "Veterinarians don't know anything about horse feet."

It's up to you to help these two get along. Most veterinarians don't shoe horses. Most horseshoers aren't veterinarians. Both are asked for their opinions about the feet of a horse. Both tend to be sure that they know how to help the horse. Both are sure that their opinions are the right ones. Unfortunately, when their opinions differ it's next to impossible to get either to change his or her mind. Egos get involved. If you can get the two people to work together, you're going to be way ahead of the game (two heads are better than one, right?).

HOOF GROWTH

The hoof wall grows from the coronary band. The sole of the foot grows from the live tissue of the sole. The frog grows from the live tissue underneath the frog. What you see on the bottom of the foot reflects something that happened a while ago because what you see on the bottom had to grow out to where it is now. All of the tissue that you can see is dead, just like your fingernail. But there's a lot of live tissue underneath the dead hoof that you can't see.

The hoof grows only about eight to ten millimeters per month, the rate of growth slower in cold or dry climates because the hoof wall tends to dry out. Because the heel of the hoof is shorter than the toe, the heels replace themselves at a quicker rate than does the toe. That is, at a steady rate of growth, the heels will replace themselves in four or five months while the toes will replace themselves in as much as twelve months. The hoof of the heels is softer and more elastic than the rest of the hoof; this is because the hoof of the heel is relatively younger than any other part of the foot.[16] The fact that the heels are softer may be one of the reasons that horses are so prone to heel problems.

When horses have hoof problems, everyone would like to be able to make the hoof grow faster, presumably so that the problem can grow out rapidly. As a result, people have come up with all sorts of great ideas on how to speed up the growth of the hoof. The only thing that these methods have in common is that none of them have been shown to work.

For instance, people will try to irritate the coronary band using mild counterirritants. Supposedly, if it were possible to increase the circulation (again) to the coronary band by irritating it, then the hoof could grow faster. The problems with this line of thinking are several. First off, no one has ever shown that applying an irritant to the coronary band will increase hoof growth. (It would be easy to show increased hoof growth if it could happen, and no one has.) Second, no one has ever shown that you can increase the circulation to the coronary band (or anywhere else). Finally, even if you could increase the circulation, why in the world would anyone think that it would cause the hoof to grow faster? Before you know it, people are going to be putting irritants on their cuticles so that their fingernails can grow faster.

THE "IMPORTANCE" OF THE FROG

The frog was given a whole lot of importance for a long time. It was said to be the pump that pushed the blood back up out of the foot. (Old horse health question: "Why does a horse have five hearts? One to move the blood in the body and four frogs to move the blood out of the feet.") Well, now veterinarians know better. The frog is a bunch of dead tissue. It doesn't pump any blood. It just sits there.[16]

That's not to say that the frog is not useful. For instance, in the author's experience, in some horses with sore soles from a variety of conditions, relief can sometimes be obtained by making the frog carry some of the weight with a pad or a shoe. (Why all the qualifications? Because this trick doesn't always work!) So the frog can be useful; it just doesn't pump blood out of the foot.

WHITE HOOVES VS. DARK HOOVES

What about horses with white feet? Aren't white feet weaker than dark feet? There's an old saying: "One white foot buy 'em, two white feet try 'em, three white feet eye 'em, four white feet shoot 'em."

Well, white feet seem to be just fine, thank you. There has actually been a study of the chemical composition of white and black hooves. There are no differences.[17]

WEAK HOOVES

If a horse's hooves are weak, can you make them stronger? You will be comforted by this answer. It appears to be yes. There have been at least two papers published on the beneficial effects of biotin on horse hooves. Biotin is a member of the A vitamin group. At a dose of fifteen to thirty milligrams per day, improvement in the quality of horse's hooves has been noted, both grossly (looking at the foot) and microscopically. (The work with biotin was first done in pigs, and then someone tried it on horses and it worked out pretty well.) Biotin supplementation apparently doesn't work all the time[18] and it does not work immediately—it takes about six months to see anything, since hoof growth starts at the top and grows down[19,20]—but biotin can help improve hoof quality. Other supplements for the hoof, like methionine and gelatin, haven't panned out, however.

What about hoof dressings? You're on your own here. No one has ever looked at them to see if they really do anything, and no one has ever compared one against the other. Nor has anyone ever done a study to see if hoof dressings can cause a hoof to retain or acquire moisture. Most horses do just fine without them. When in doubt, always fall back on the "horses are like cars" analogy.

HOOF ABSCESSES

A hoof abscess occurs when an area of the foot becomes infected. When the cause can be established, this point of infection is frequently related to a previous penetrating wound, for example, a nail.[21] Sometimes the cause can't be established.

Abscesses are made up of pus, a liquid that forms from the body's response to whatever caused the problem in the first place. In the hoof, the formation of pus is a particular pain because the liquid has nowhere to go when it forms. The hoof is a hard, fairly rigid structure. Therefore, as the abscess expands, pressure builds up within the foot because the foot can't stretch. The increase in pressure underneath the hoof wall causes pain. The horse with a growing abscess becomes more and more lame because he absolutely does not want to put any weight on something that hurts as much as his hoof does. Consequently, abscesses are one of the more dramatic forms of lameness in the horse. Horses with foot abscesses can look like they have broken their legs, which, of course, causes various degrees of hysteria in horse owners.

Fortunately, hoof abscesses are usually easily corrected. The abscess can generally be located rather easily when it is prodded with a hoof-testing device or with a hoof knife. Once the abscessed area is located, the infection is opened up and allowed to drain. After a few days the horse will almost always be fine.

There are two lessons to be learned from this. The first is that if your horse was fine last night and is really lame today, look at the foot first (unless there's something really obvious, like protruding bone). You may not be able see anything, but if the horse is really lame and it comes up quickly, chances are that the foot is the culprit. An abscess of the hoof is not an uncommon occurrence.

To treat an abscess, people will have you soaking the foot and wrapping it with a variety of medications. It is very useful to keep an open area of the bottom of the foot clean and bandaged to keep manure and dirt out of it while the tissue heals. All the soaking that is done to "draw out" abscesses probably just works to rinse out the foot. Once you recognize the problem, most hoof abscesses will take care of themselves.

A gravel is a hoof abscess that comes out at the coronary band instead of the bottom of the hoof. As an abscess grows, it expands toward the point of least resistance. If the abscess occurs high in the hoof wall, that point may be the coronary band.

A gravel has nothing to do with gravel, that is, crushed rock. This condition got its name because a small piece of gravel supposedly enters the bottom of the hoof and works its way out the top, but this isn't what happens at all. A gravel is just a hoof abscess with a colorful name.

THRUSH

Thrush is an infection of the foot. The infection eats away at the hoof tissue. Thrush is smelly and gooey and stinky (medical terms, all) and it almost always is found in the crevices of the frog (the sulci) or between the heels. These are the areas that are the most difficult to clean and the areas in which dirt and manure can most easily accumulate.

Thrush is usually caused by some sort of bacteria. The type of bacteria isn't at all important, since it is undoubtedly one of a smorgasbord of bacteria that exist in the ground of wherever your horse lives. If your horse has thrush, there will be a moist, smelly and painful area of his hoof. Usually thrush is relatively easy to control, but if it goes unrecognized, it can eat through the hard tissues of the foot and get into the sensitive structures below.[22]

Thrush is not the white stuff that you see on the bottom of the sole when you are cleaning the foot. Nor is thrush the peeling of the sole and/or frog that you sometimes begin to see when the horse is overdue for trimming. It is natural for the sole and frog to peel off, just like a callous on your hand. Nor do all smelly feet have thrush. When a pad is taken off a horse's foot, you will experience the pungent smell of the bacteria that have grown in the moist environment that the pad caused, but that doesn't mean there's thrush. (It is true that pads on a horse's foot can cause the sole to soften, although this does not necessarily cause the horse any problems.) Finally, thrush is not contagious, that is, it can't be spread among a group of horses by using a hoof pick, for example.

Thrush is easily prevented by keeping the horse's foot clean and the bedding dry. An ounce of prevention really is worth a pound of cure. The cures are legion, however.

There are probably hundreds of treatments for thrush. Most involve squirting or packing all sorts of noxious substances into the foot, in addition to keeping the feet clean. It may also be necessary to trim out some of the infected tissue with a hoof knife.[22] Treatment is tedious, but it does work eventually. Remember, if you just work on keeping your horse's feet clean and dry in the first place, you won't have to worry much about thrush.

INTERNAL HOOF PROBLEMS

Problems with the interior of the hoof can be terribly frustrating for everyone involved. While external problems like abscesses and thrush are relatively easy to recognize and treat, veterinary science has yet to come up with a way to look inside the horse's hoof and accurately determine all of the problems that can occur there. This point comes up again and again. Patience and "tincture of time" are frequently the most valuable treatments for problems that involve the internal structures of the hoof.

How to sum this up? Well, carefully. Science doesn't know very much about what happens to horse's hooves when they are messed with by trimming and shoeing. The results that are predicted may not always be the results that are obtained. Unfortunately, a bit of trial and error always ends up being the only consistent method of obtaining a good end result. Good hoof care on your part will do wonders to prevent any serious medical problems. But just because you try to do things for your horse by the book doesn't mean that he's going to read it.

15

Navicular Disease
(The Big Myth)

It is time to discuss one of the most overdiagnosed, overinterpreted, over-treated and overexposed conditions of the horse. Navicular disease is not what you think.

What is the navicular bone, anyway? It is a bone (naturally) that lies within the horse's hoof in the heel region. It is a very important bone. The tendon of the deep flexor muscle runs right over the top of this bone. The tendon makes a turn around the navicular bone and then attaches to the bone of the foot (the coffin bone). As the horse strides and the foot hits the ground, tremendous stress is applied to the heel area.[1] When the flexor muscles contract, they pull the foot up and off the ground via the tendons. The navicular bone may help with this lifting by serving as a fulcrum for the tendon of the deep flexor muscle. (A fulcrum is a turning point for a lever. If you are trying to pry a rock up out of the ground with a bar, your work is made much easier if you put a rock or something underneath the bar, so that you can pry against it. In this example, the rock is a fulcrum.) The navicular bone is, therefore, an important stress point for the horse.

The horse's heel takes a pretty heavy beating in the course of a normal day. Most of the horse's weight is carried on the front end (approximately 60 percent in the standing horse),[2] and at the trot the force on the front legs is 35 to 40 percent greater than on the back legs![3] It is no wonder that the majority of lameness problems occur in the front feet.[4,5] The feet pound into the ground with each stride, and when the horse strides, the heels, especially the inside (medial) heel, take most of the impact.[6] The heels are also the softest part of the foot and the part nearest the ground.[7] It will therefore come as no surprise that many of the front foot problems in the horse occur in the heels. Not all heel problems, however, involve the navicular bone.

There are a lot of important structures in the heel of the horse's foot besides the navicular bone, including bones, ligaments, tendon and joints.[8] Any of these structures can be injured, and to the examiner it's often impossible to distinguish between injuries to the various structures. Unfortunately, there are severe limitations to a veterinarian's abilities to identify individual structures in the heel area. Consequently, a lot of the injuries to other structures in the heels get lumped together under the heading of navicular disease.

NAVICULAR DISEASE VS. NAVICULAR SYNDROME

To add to all the confusion, there's not even much of a consensus on what to call problems associated with the navicular area. "True" navicular disease is supposed to refer to a deterioration of the navicular bone. "Disease" seems to imply that there is a single cause and a single cure; nothing could be further from the truth about this condition. Many veterinarians prefer to use the term "navicular syndrome" to refer to problems of the navicular bone and its associated structures, the ligaments of the bone and the deep flexor tendon.[9] "Syndrome" does allow veterinarians to lump more things under one name, but it unfortunately adds one more term to the overall confusion about just exactly what is going on.

When most people think of "navicular," they are usually thinking of a bad problem for the horse. When navicular bone deterioration does occur in the navicular syndrome, it is generally progressive and it frequently does not respond well to treatment. Its cause is unknown.

THE SIGNS OF NAVICULAR DISEASE

When navicular disease occurs, it is most commonly in both front feet. It almost always affects the front feet, although the hind feet can rarely be affected. The disease generally develops slowly and becomes chronic. It is difficult, if not impossible, to reverse.

Navicular disease is a disease of horses seven to fourteen years old. This is probably because these horses are out there performing and stressing their heels. Horses less than three years and more than fifteen years old are three to five times less likely to develop navicular disease than are the seven- to fourteen-year-olds.[10] Chances are, if your horse is very young or very old, he's not going to have navicular problems. Keep this in mind if your young or old horse develops sore heels.

Navicular disease can be a damning diagnosis for your horse. If your horse does have navicular disease, you may be in for a lot of frustration. The ideal goal of curing the condition is not one that can always be attained, particularly after secondary changes involving the ligaments and deep flexor tendon set in (the more advanced cases).[11] No one wants to own a horse that has navicular disease, and everyone wants to try to identify a horse that has it, particularly before they own it. Unfortunately, for reasons that you will see, this is not possible. That does not, however, stop people from trying to aggressively identify any horse that does or might have the condition. This leads, inevitably, to mistaken and overeager diagnosis.

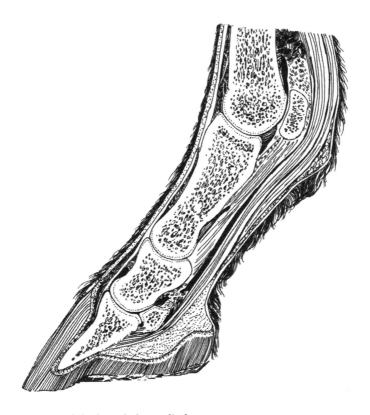

Complex anatomy of the horse's lower limb.

THE RISKS OF OVERDIAGNOSIS

Navicular disease is most likely overdiagnosed for two reasons. First, other than the coffin bone, it is the only one of the many structures in the heel area that veterinarians can see using diagnostic imaging techniques. Since veterinarians can see it, they can easily comment on it. One of the real limitations of equine medicine today is that veterinarians cannot look inside the hoof very effectively. Other structures besides the bone may be injured; they just can't be identified using currently available methods of diagnosis. A horse may tear the impar ligament of the navicular bone, for example, but there is no way that *any* veterinarian could tell you this with assurance.

Second, navicular disease is overdiagnosed because it apparently satisfies people's lamentable tendency to give a name to something. People just will not be happy unless a condition has a name. "Heel soreness" must not be a very satisfying name to most people. But, if instead of "heel soreness," the horse is said to have "navicular syndrome," people will have a condition with a catchy name to discuss. They may not know what it is but at least it has a name.

This is a well-recognized phenomenon. James Herriot, the best-selling English veterinarian/author, was advised by another practitioner to give every condition a name. "Call it McCluskey's disease," call it anything, but at least give your client something to call the problem. It's sort of a badge of honor.

"My horse has navicular," says the owner.

"Too bad," says his/her friend, shaking his/her head.

Together, they sympathize and bond.

Because navicular disease is such a bad diagnosis for the horse, it behooves you, as the horse owner, to make sure that a diagnosis is made carefully and thoughtfully. You should never say "navicular disease" casually.

DIAGNOSIS

Navicular disease cannot be diagnosed by the way a horse's foot looks. You can't look at a horse and say, "Now there's a horse that's going to have problems with his navicular bones." In fact, veterinarians can't seem to agree on what the most likely foot to develop navicular disease looks like. Ask U. S. veterinarians and they will tell you about a big Quarter Horse with little teeny contracted and upright feet. Ask European veterinarians and they will tell you about a big platter-footed warmblood with no heel. Although veterinarians tend to associate disease of the navicular bones with a particular foot conformation, if that conformation exists it does not assure that the horse will develop a problem in the navicular area.

The history of your horse's lameness is very important in making the diagnosis of navicular disease. Navicular is insidious and usually does not occur all of a sudden. It creeps up on your horse. Over time, you may notice that your horse starts to get a bit of a short stride. You may notice that he limps only on tight turns. You may notice that the condition gets gradually worse. You may find that the condition affects both legs—it almost always does[10,11]—that he doesn't turn well in *either* direction. You will worry. If your horse was fine yesterday and very lame today, however, he almost certainly does *not* have navicular disease.

The diagnosis of navicular disease must be arrived at very carefully. The diagnosis of heel soreness is relatively easy to come to for your veterinarian. The difficulty with making the diagnosis of navicular disease is that there are no clear-cut and reliable steps that can be used to verify a diagnosis or separate it from all of the other causes of heel soreness. Here are some of the things that are commonly used in the diagnosis of the condition.

LAMENESS AS SIGN

A horse with navicular disease must be lame. This is such an obvious requirement for a proper diagnosis of this condition that it is astonishing that it is frequently overlooked. *If the horse is not lame, he doesn't have navicular disease.* And he doesn't have "pre-navicular" disease because there is no such thing. You can't predict if a horse is going to develop navicular disease.

HOOF TESTERS

The "navicular" horse will hopefully (from a diagnostic standpoint) show some sensitivity in his heels. Most commonly, horses with navicular disease will show some sensitivity when hoof testers are applied with one jaw across the frog and the other jaw on the opposing hoof wall. If, when the hoof testers are squeezed together, the resulting pressure causes the horse pain, the horse will typically try to pull his foot away from the source of pain (wouldn't you?). Not all horses show hoof-tester sensitivity in this fashion, however.

STRESS TESTS

The horse with navicular disease may show some increased soreness to various stress tests. For instance, if you hold a horse's leg up in the air and flex him at the fetlock joint for, say, sixty seconds, he may, if he has sore heels, limp more dramatically than before flexion. This could be because he doesn't want to drop his sore foot down on the ground. It may also be because flexing the leg squishes all the tissue in the lower part of the leg together. (It could be from another problem higher up in the leg.) And he may not limp at all after such a test. Other stress tests, such as standing the horse on an angled block of wood followed by immediate trotting, may also be helpful (or not) in sorting out heel soreness.[11]

REGIONAL ANESTHETICS

The most commonly used test in the diagnosis of navicular disease is the use of regional anesthesia. Two big nerves run down to the heel area along the back of the pastern, on either side of the deep flexor tendon. *In addition to everything else in the heel,* these nerves supply the navicular bone. You can feel the area where they are located on the back of the pastern, right alongside the two big arteries that run along either side of the prominent deep flexor tendon. If you place a small amount of anesthetic over the nerves, the heels go numb. If the horse is limping because his heels hurt, he will stop limping when they are numb. *All this test does is show that the soreness comes from some tissue that is found in the heels.* It does not mean that the soreness comes from the navicular bone. Unfortunately, many veterinarians will diagnose any lameness that improves following local anesthetic block as navicular.[11]

Most horses with navicular disease are sore in both front feet. One of the most commonly made observations is that when a navicular horse's heels are made numb in the leg on which he is most obviously limping, he will then begin to limp noticeably on the other leg. It is not always possible to observe that a horse is limping on both front feet simultaneously, especially if one foot hurts more than the other. When the soreness is relieved in the one foot, however, the horse feels only the pain in the other foot and thus "switches" his lameness to the other leg that now is the most prominent source of pain. Just because the horse shows lameness in both feet doesn't mean that he has disease of the navicular bone.

X RAYS

As a concluding part of the routine diagnostic process, X rays may be taken. Now a can of worms opens.

There have been some very elegant studies done involving X rays of the navicular bone. In these studies, X rays of clinically normal horses are compared to those of horses that have been diagnosed with navicular disease. The results? In one study, 60 percent of normal horses had "changes" in their navicular bones consistent with navicular disease, compared with 70 percent of the horses that had been diagnosed as having the problem.[12]

In addition, a number of variations in the X ray appearance of the shape and consistency of the navicular bone was noted in a study conducted on over five hundred normal horses.[13] Some of these variations are the same types of things that are consistently diagnosed as a problem in other horses.

You have to look at navicular changes in one of two ways. Maybe there are a whole bunch of horses running around just waiting to develop navicular disease, since so many normal horses have "changes." Or maybe navicular bone X rays aren't all that great at telling if a horse really has problems in that area.

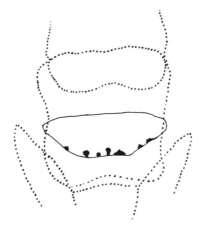

The navicular bone (solid line) as it appears on an X ray. The black spots are "changes." The "changes" shown here could be normal but could also be interpreted as abnormal, depending on who's interpreting.

The truth is, a veterinarian can't tell if a horse has navicular disease just by looking at his X rays. Some horses with normal navicular bone X rays have disease of the navicular bone. Some horses with horrible navicular bone X rays will never be lame. Nobody knows why this is so, but apparently X rays do not reflect the actual state of the navicular bone's health. And most especially, no one can *ever* predict if a horse is *going* to develop navicular disease in the future by looking at X rays.[14]

Sadly, a lot of horses get condemned (or turned down on prepurchase evaluations) because of navicular bone "changes" on X rays. When veterinarians look at a navicular bone, they all seem to be able to agree on what a normal navicular bone looks like, that is, when it is free of any variations from the ideal. In some horses, changes show up on the X rays. These changes may appear as little holes in the bone or irregularities at the corners or along the edges. (Some veterinarians have given the changes colorful names like "lollipops"). These changes may reflect some past damage to the navicular bone, but they also may not. X ray changes in the navicular bone do not correspond well to deterioration of the bone.[9] Navicular bone changes may only be mere variations from normal.

What is a normal variation?

Take your feet, for example. Let's say that you stand with your feet slightly turned out. Your friend stands with her feet slightly turned in. What's normal? You both are normal (with any luck). You just differ.

In the same manner, X ray changes on a navicular bone don't necessarily indicate a problem. X rays show normal variations between individuals. Abnormal navicular bone X rays don't mean that a horse has or will develop a problem with the navicular bone.

Wouldn't it be nice if you could predict that a horse was going to have navicular disease? Many people do. They do so in error.

So what good are X rays?

In some horses, if all the clinical signs are right, X rays can be a useful diagnostic tool. They can be an important bit of evidence in the diagnosis of the problems underlying sore heels. In a lame horse that is sore to hoof testers in the right area, that has a bad response to certain stress tests, that is sound on one leg after heel anesthesia and switches lameness to the other leg and is then sound on that leg after heel anesthesia, "abnormal" X rays may provide a bit of extra evidence that the navicular bone may be the source of a horse's lameness.[10,11] But in and of themselves, X rays are basically worthless.

Interpretative variation is another very important thing to be aware of, especially in the diagnosis of navicular disease. Let's say you are asked, "Is that a pretty song?" The answer may be obvious to you if you love the song, but someone else may not like the song at all. Those sorts of differences are interpretative variations. They are influenced highly by experience and personal philosophy.

Because of interpretative variation, it is possible for two people, even two "experts," to differ widely in their assessment of the same thing. In the case of navicular disease, this means that two veterinarians can come to completely different conclusions from examining the same set of scintigraphic scans (or X rays, for that matter).

SCINTIGRAPHY

So if you go through all of the aforementioned diagnostics, you know what? You still may not know for sure if your horse has navicular disease.

Therefore, techniques other than X rays are being employed in the diagnosis of navicular disease. Scintigraphy, which is discussed in the first chapter, is one of them. Scintigraphy is best used in conjunction with X rays, to help support X ray changes (if they exist) or to aid in locating a problem if X rays are normal.[15] Scintigraphy can give you some indication that the heel area is inflamed.[16]

Scintigraphy will not, however, tell you about the changes inside the foot, and it cannot tell you if there are any problems with the ligaments or tendons because it cannot directly image these structures. Scintigraphy is very sensitive; unfortunately, it may also be associated with some horses being falsely identified as having inflammation in the heel area.[15] It may be able to give you some idea if there is some inflammation in the bone of the heel or in the soft tissue, although this is full of interpretive variation (as is scintigraphy in general).

It should now be apparent to you that there is at least a possibility that your horse with sore heels may not have navicular disease after all. This may be a source of some comfort, although it is potentially quite confusing, without doubt. It is completely within the realm of possibility that your horse can be abnormal on all of the diagnostic tests used to demonstrate navicular disease and still not have the condition.

Therefore, some authorities say that a diagnosis of navicular disease should not be made unless a horse fails to respond to a variety of treatments for heel soreness for several months.[9] This, of course, requires considerable patience and understanding (and cash) on your part, and unfortunately some owners have not been given a generous supply of these qualities. Remember this: Navicular disease is the first diagnosis of the diagnostically destitute and the last diagnosis of a careful diagnostician.

TREATMENT

Given the difficulties in diagnosis, it only makes sense that treatment for navicular disease is on some kind of trial-and-error basis. Treatment is not always easy and it may not always be successful.

The whole idea in treating horses with heel soreness (and navicular disease) is to try to relieve the pain in the heel and, ideally, to correct the underlying problem, right? In attempts to do this, veterinarians can:

1. Use drugs to cover up the pain. It's not very therapeutic, but sometimes it's the best you can do.
2. Protect the heels with some sort of horseshoe. Some people report very successful results using an egg bar shoe (which is slightly different from a regular or D bar shoe in that the bar extends back behind the heels).[17] Other people feel that this sort of shoe is not at all helpful.

3. Protect and cushion the heels by elevating them with a pad.[18,19]

    Some people feel that elevating the heels with a pad may have a beneficial effect by relaxing some strain to the deep flexor tendon and ligaments of the pastern and navicular bone. (This effect of horseshoeing was discussed in the chapter on hooves.)

4. Change the way that the foot is trimmed in an effort to relieve pressure from here or there; correct any obvious problems and decrease the work of moving the foot.[11,19]

    There is no reason why you couldn't combine principles of numbers 2, 3 and 4. This would imply that all horses should be shod according to their individual needs, as opposed to doing it by some stock formula. (That's not a bad idea.)

5. Try to affect the circulation to the foot. This is based on the idea that circulation problems in the foot are associated with the development of navicular disease.

Isoxsuprine hydrochloride is a drug that is commonly prescribed to improve or increase the circulation to the horse's foot by dilating small blood vessels. No one, unfortunately, has even demonstrated that the drug does what it claims to, but it does seem to help some horses with navicular disease.[11,20,21]

Only one carefully controlled study has been done on the response of horses with navicular disease to treatment with isoxsuprine. Horses with navicular responded positively to isoxsuprine while those that were treated with a placebo (a nondrug pill) showed no effect, as would be expected.[21]

That's the good news.

However, if some isoxsuprine is good, more is not necessarily better. In the same study, there was no beneficial effect to be had from increasing the dose of the drug. This suggests that if your horse doesn't respond to the normal doses of this drug, giving him more won't help. (Another study couldn't detect *any* levels of the drug in the horse's serum when it was given at recommended doses.)[11]

Furthermore, there was absolutely no correlation among X-ray evidence of navicular disease, the degree of lameness and the response to treatment.[21] This means that if your horse has navicular disease, there is no way to tell in advance if he is going to respond to treatment with this drug.

The consensus of opinion now is that circulation problems in the foot don't seem to cause navicular disease anyway.[9,10,11] Consequently, the pharmacologic basis for using isoxsuprine may not be valid! The drug works in some horses anyway.

6. Give local injections into the heels to try to relieve inflammation.[22] Though difficult, injections of cortisone into the navicular bursa, which cushions the deep flexor tendon as it runs over the navicular bone, have provided some relief for some horses. The relief is usually short-lived, however, and long-term results of this treatment are thought to be effective in less than 5 percent of the horses treated in this manner.[11]

7. Perform surgery. Cutting the nerves to the foot takes away the pain in the heels for a while. This procedure, called "nerving," is usually done as a last resort. Basically you're sweeping the horse's problem under the rug. You can't fix it, so you cover it up. You can prolong a horse's useful life by this procedure, but the underlying problems in the heel will continue.[10,11]

   All sorts of myths exist about the denerving procedure. The denerving procedure is not dangerous for the horse; the surgeon is only cutting the nerves to the heel. The horse retains sensation in the rest of the foot after denerving and will be able to feel where his foot is and should not stumble or be unsafe. Complications can occur as a result of this surgery (as with any surgery). Discuss them with your veterinarian before considering this operation.[9,10,11]

   Unfortunately, the nerves will grow back together after a denerving procedure (yes, nerves do grow). The horse will reestablish feeling in his heels when this happens. Approximately 60 percent of the horses will go two years before the nerves come back, according to the studies.[23] But nerving may ultimately be the only way to add *any* years to your horse's performing life if his condition cannot be relieved by medicine, rest or shoeing.

   Other surgeries are described for the treatment of navicular disease, such as cutting the suspensory ligaments of the navicular bone[24] and fasciotomy (dissection of the nerves to free them up from the surrounding tissue).[25] Though some preliminary results of these surgeries have been promising, no one knows how to pick the horses that might benefit from such surgeries, and some complications have been seen. A lot more work needs to be done before these surgeries can be routinely recommended.[26]

8. Try a variety of home and old Indian remedies. This is not therapy; it's desperation.

The biggest myth about navicular disease, in the author's opinion, is that it is the most common lameness affecting horses. It may be one of the most commonly *diagnosed,* however. In fact, many horses that are unjustly condemned as having navicular disease may be able to return to normal function with some time and treatment. Just because your horse has sore heels, just because his

X rays aren't normal and just because your next door neighbor says so, doesn't mean that your horse has navicular disease.

Navicular disease is a particularly difficult problem, both in diagnosis and treatment. You should try a variety of treatments for sore heels before deciding that your horse may have disease of the navicular bone. A veterinarian's ability to accurately diagnose problems in the heel area is quite limited, and he or she may not be able to tell you exactly what your horse's problem is with any degree of certainty. Because of this, you should work closely and, above all, patiently with your veterinarian and farrier to try to come up with a solution to your horse's heel problem. Many horses can have heel problems that are not navicular disease and that can also take many, many months to resolve. Many horses with navicular disease can be helped, at least temporarily.[11]

Anyone who looks at your horse and casually says "Looks like your horse could have a touch of navicular" is a bit touched. Don't throw your horse, or any horse, in the wastebasket diagnosis that navicular disease has become.

PART VI

MISCELLANY

16

Behavior

Why do horses do the things they do? Unfortunately, you can't ask them. (Well, you can but they won't answer.) The answer to the question is "Nobody knows." Most people are not satisfied with that answer. Consequently, they follow a time-honored tradition. If people don't know the reason, they make it up. Frequently, it becomes dogma.

When horses are observed, the observers note how they act in certain situations and try to associate those actions with events that occur before or during those situations. For instance, every time a certain horse sees a big truck, he goes nuts. What is *known* is that this occurs. You still don't know why. Does he not like trucks? How about truck drivers? Does the noise bother him? Did he have a bad experience being hauled? These sorts of questions are unanswerable without the complete, detailed knowledge of the horse's past history that is generally not available to the observer.

Horses are relatively predictable, particularly as individuals. Once you get to know a horse, you can expect certain behaviors. Horses are creatures of habit. They like to be fed the same thing, all the time (no Cajun food for them, please) at regular intervals. These are rather timid creatures, in spite of their size. They feel safe and secure in their stalls (even if they are a bit confining), even in the face of danger. This is thought to be why horses run back into their barns during a fire, for example.

It is odd that so many people are afraid of horses. Although they are big, they are not at all mean. And horses are not generally aggressive.[1] When they see something they don't recognize, their first instinct is to run from it. They aren't very well equipped to fight, although they do have weapons like teeth and hooves. They would prefer to run from something and then try to figure out

179

what it is from a distance. Knowing this, you might be able to predict that a horse would demonstrate behaviors like spooking or shying at unknown objects or sounds from time to time. How much a particular horse spooks, however, is a matter of the horse's personality and training.

Horses in the wild are, of course, herd animals. They like being with other horses. In the wild, horses usually travel in social groups called harems, made up of one male, several adult females and their offspring, which are usually less than three years old. Horses are not at all territorial and groups wander about the countryside, but the stallions are very protective of their group. There are also bachelor bands made up of those stallions that aren't lucky enough to have a harem. Bachelors are looking for opportunities to take over another

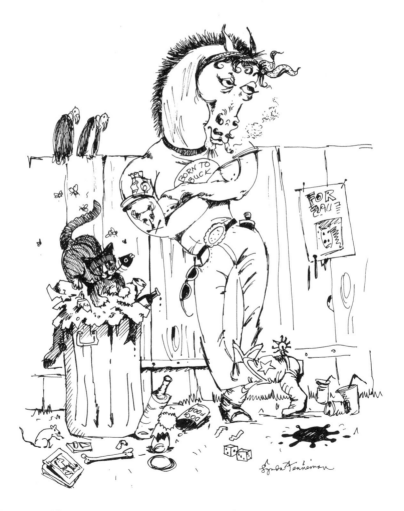

The signs of bad behavior should be recognized early.

stallion's harem or start their own. Harems are stable social units, and most of the coming and going from them is done by the youngsters in the group.[2]

Life being what it is, most people are somehow unable to keep a herd of horses on large tracts of land. Because of this, horses are usually kept in conditions that they are not normally or naturally in. This eliminates two significant characteristics of a horse's normal and natural life. That is, they live in small, confined spaces, separated from other horses, and they are fed twice a day, as opposed to being able to graze constantly in groups.

You can take the horse out of nature, but the nature of the horse cannot be taken out of him. Horses are gregarious, active and curious. Kept in the abnormal circumstances that are forced on them, it's no wonder that horses develop habits. The poor things are probably bored to tears.

STALL VICES

Stall vices, like crib biting (cribbing), teeth rubbing, stall walking and stall weaving, are apparently things that the horse learns to do to pass the time. These habits are pretty annoying if you watch the horse do them for a while. But "vice" implies that the horses are somehow immoral for performing these behaviors and that they would stop if they only had the willpower. It's pretty clear that these behaviors are developed by the horse as a way to help him cope with his abnormal environment.[3] Horses develop habits in the stall to help pass the time.

"Vices" don't really cause much harm to the horse. Not that they don't bother the horse owners. They make horse owners crazy! Cribbing, for instance, is considered by some people to be an unsoundness. This really isn't justified. Here's another myth to break.

CRIBBING

Cribbing is a behavior characterized by the horse biting firmly onto an object and pulling back while at the same time sucking air into his mouth. Cribbing is *not* a result of domestication. Horses in the wild have been observed to crib. Cribbers latch on to any piece of metal or wood, pull back and "suck wind" for all they are worth.[3]

The biggest problem with cribbing is that the horse can wear down his front teeth at an alarming pace. Before you know it, your horse can have a set of upper teeth that look just like a cow's (none there). Since he doesn't have to graze if he's kept in a stall, however, that doesn't present him with any huge problems.

It's a myth that when horses suck wind they swallow huge amounts of air. This air, supposedly, stretches the stomach or intestines and makes the horse colic. Sorry, but it doesn't seem to be so. There just aren't any demonstrably bad effects from cribbing.[3] For that reason, all of the things that are done to try to stop horses from cribbing, like collars and electric wires and surgery, seem somehow less important. Cribbers may drive you nuts. But unless an otherwise healthy horse is losing weight because he cribs all the time or can be demonstrated to have a *problem* with air ingestion, it's not worth the effort to try to stop him.

People generally assume that if one horse in the barn develops a habit like cribbing or stall weaving, then the other horses in the barn will learn to do so rapidly and pretty soon there will be a whole barn of horses swaying rhythmically together like human heads at a tennis match. This has never been proven, however. It is possible that the environment that causes one horse to develop a stall vice may also cause another one to do the same thing.[3]

While it's pretty clear that horses develop stall vices due to boredom, it's also clear that, at least in the case of cribbing, horses do it because it makes them feel good. In horses (and us, too) the body manufactures a group of chemicals known as endorphins. These natural substances are very similar to narcotics. They produce a sensation of euphoria. It has been shown that when a horse cribs, higher levels of these chemicals are found in the blood. When a drug is given to the horse that blocks the effects of narcotics, horses tend to crib much less.[4] Apparently, horses crib because an endorphin release makes them high.

(As an aside, it's also interesting that the endorphin release also appears to be why a nose twitch works as a restraint device. The blocking drug keeps a twitch from working, as well. Some people feel that a nose twitch is actually a type of acupuncture.[5] Twitches apparently do not work as restraint devices because they cause pain.)

CHEWING WOOD

Horses love to chew wood, too. Some of them seem to be related to beavers. This is another irritating thing that they do, particularly since wood is such a convenient and readily available source of material to keep horses confined with. Horses actually eat the wood, even though they can't digest it. Although wood chewing has been associated with a lack of roughage in the diet of horses fed grains or pellets,[6] wild horses are known to eat trees and shrubs, too.[7] It may be that horses need some indigestible fiber in their diet. Horses may also be motivated to chew through the side of a stall to try to get to a neighbor and chat.[3] As with cribbing, wood chewing is another habit that isn't harmful to the horse.

"CURING" THE STALL VICE PROBLEM

The ideal way to try to cure the problems of stable vices is to give the horse something to do. Allowing a horse access to a larger space, when possible, can help reduce boredom. So can giving him toys or providing him a companion, like a goat or a sheep. Increased frequency of feeding or increased amounts of a lower-calorie hay may help the horse pass the time in his stall by eating.[3] However, all of the attention, aggravation and effort that is given to the control of stall vices is probably just not worth it.

DOMINANCE

Much of horse behavior can be explained by recognizing the phenomenon of dominance. In the wild, whenever two horses live together, one will be dominant over the other. The simplest form of dominance is shown by a horse moving in and taking over another horse's space. Upon first meeting, horses may display aggression toward each other, and one will withdraw. Aggressive horses will lay their ears back and threaten to bite, strike or kick, but they rarely carry these threats out. While establishing dominance, horses rarely hurt each other. Aggression that is actually carried out has a high cost to the group of horses in terms of injury to herd members, increased energy expenditure and disruption of normal herd behavior.[2] As a result, one horse will establish dominance over the other.

Dominance relationships are stable. While adult horses tend to dominate young horses, what factors influence dominance are not at all clear. Sex, height and weight are apparently not important factors. Disposition and temperament do seem to be important because smaller, younger and aggressive horses tend to reach higher social rank than do older, more passive, larger horses.[2]

In unnatural situations, like pastures and stalls, dominance relationships will still try to be established. Of special importance is the relationship that the horse has with his owner. While most horses are passive and will allow owners to come in, halter them, brush them and perform all sorts of other weird "owner" behaviors, some horses will resent these intrusions and try to prevent their occurrence. As such, it is very important for the owner of the horse to not allow the horse to begin to dominate the relationship.

While this may mean that striking the horse is necessary to punish a negative behavior, ultimately the rewards of having a more submissive horse far outweigh the potential danger of having a twelve-hundred-pound animal that thinks he runs the show.

It is a myth that hitting a horse is always a mean and uncalled-for act. There's never an excuse for beating a horse into a frenzy, but an aggressive show of dominance on the part of the owner or trainer is language a horse can understand.

COMMUNICATION

Horses communicate with each other freely. No one knows, of course, what they are saying, but relationships have been observed between certain types of communication and behavior. To communicate, horses make use of their senses of sight, sense, touch and smell as well as their ability to vocalize. People have to learn how to communicate with horses since they can't figure out how to talk to people.

VOCALIZATION

Vocalizations are common in horses. Horses often respond to threats of aggression with a brief, high-pitched squeal. A lower-pitched, quiet sound (nicker) is generally a sound of contentment (and absolutely heartwarming to hear). It occurs in wild horses when the stallion is courting the mare, when the mare is calling the foal or when the foal approaches his mother.[2] In stabled horses, you'll hear lots of nickering around feeding time. Whinnying or neighing, the louder, more familiar sounds that horses make, are anxious sounds. Mares and foals will whinny when they have lost sight of each other. Foals can distinguish the whinny of their mother.[2] Whinnying appears to be a more long-range (and louder) form of communication. Blowing air through the nostrils (snorting), though not vocal, is another audible form of communication. It is generally a sign of alarm or a reaction to an unrecognized object.[2]

SMELL

Communication through the sense of smell is less well understood in horses. Mares sniff and smell their newborn foals. This forms an important and distinctly recognizable bond between them. When horses first meet, they sniff noses, flank and rear to gain information as to the identity (and possibly determine the reproductive status of) each other.[2] Some horses seem to sense the smell of disinfectants on the hands of veterinarians and react with fright. Much about communication through smell is not understood.

TOUCHING

Horses do love to touch and be touched. The sense of touch is very important for communication between them. Horses groom each other in the wild and many enjoy grooming by their owner. Mares and foals are in constant contact and not just when nursing.[2]

Take advantage of the fact that horses like to be touched. When moving around a horse in a stall, try to keep a hand on him or stay close against him. He will like it and generally respond positively. He will also know where you are so you will be less likely to get mashed into the side of the stall if he moves.

BODY LANGUAGE

Body parts can tell you a lot about how the horse is feeling, especially the ears. Erect and forward ears show that a horse is alert or interested. Ears that bend out to the side mean that an animal is resting or submissive. Ears that are laid back against the head signify aggression and a potential threat. Similarly, the tail, if it is raised, indicates confidence or excitement, while a tail tucked tight against the body can mean submission, fear, or just rest.[2]

INTELLIGENCE AND LEARNING

Horses are generally given credit for some intelligence, usually depending upon how the person who is doing the crediting feels about the animal at the particular time that the credit is given. For instance, as you watch your horse go bucking off into the distance after having deposited you on the ground, you will be less inclined to credit his intelligence than if he were performing one of his cute behaviors at the stall. Horses *are* intelligent and have the capability to learn. They are not rational, however; that is, they do not analyze situations and respond. They learn behaviors and repeat them or they act by instinct. It's a myth, however, and it's wrong to think that horses are completely stupid.

Knowing how horses learn is important in understanding the behavior of horses in general and helps them to be taught in a manner in which they *can* learn. It can also help you understand how behavior problems develop and give you clues as to how to solve them. Sometimes learning is intentional, that is, horses learn something that people try to teach them. Sometimes horses learn things almost accidentally because they are amazingly observant and have good memories. The two most common ways that horses learn are called habituation and conditioning.[8]

HABITUATION

Habituation is one of the simplest types of learning. This is the type of learning that results in horses adapting to (getting used to) their environment. For instance, in young horses, a variety of stimuli may make them run in fear. As horses grow older and habituate, things like blankets, leaves and barking dogs lose their ability to scare. The common practice of sacking out a young horse to get him used to stuff hanging all over his body is a good example of habituation.

If a horse stops seeing something that he is habituated to, it is possible that he will react again when exposed to it. In that way, horses do seem to forget something that they knew about before. A horse may also react to a habituated response if he reacts to another stimulus first.[8] For example, let's say that your horse no longer jumps away from dogs running at a fence as you ride by. If, however, there is a bright yellow tarp on the ground (you know how menacing those can be), the horse may react if he has not been habituated. If, after that reaction, a dog runs up and starts barking, the horse may run from that as well, sort of as part of the overall program or reaction. The first reaction can therefore override the previously habituated response.

Practically, the more often that a horse is exposed to a strange stimulus, the more quickly he will become habituated to it. Also, the more he is exposed to it, the less likely he will be to forget it. This means that for training purposes, you should repeat the exposure to a stimulus many times during a training session and repeat the exposure on other occasions when you are working with the horse. Often, during training, once a horse has responded correctly, the training is stopped. It would seem more reasonable, given their learning patterns, that insisting that the horse repeat his response several times (and congratulating him each time) would be a more appropriate method of training.[8]

CONDITIONING

Conditioning refers to an association between a stimulus and a response. There was a very famous horse at around the turn of the century named Clever Hans. His master was sure that he had taught him how to perform complex feats of arithmetic. The horse would indicate an answer by pawing the ground until the correct answer was obtained and would even answer questions from independent questioners. This marvelous animal was unmasked when it was finally observed that his master would anxiously (and unconsciously) lean forward when Hans started to answer and relax and lean back when the correct answer was reached. The horse observed that when his master leaned back, it was all right to stop pawing. Once that was discovered, Hans stopped pawing and his master lost a meal ticket.[9]

Conditioning allows a horse to learn cause-and-effect relationships between his behaviors and stimuli in his surroundings.[8] This is not, of course, always positive. Horses are tremendously observant and may become conditioned to things that you are not even aware of.

Here's a great example. You walk into the stall. Your horse turns his rear end to you and lifts his hind leg. You get him a carrot and he turns around and lets you halter him. Day after day the problem gets worse.

You may be training your horse to lift his leg up and threaten you so that he can have a carrot before he gets haltered. Or is he training you?

See, horses are not *that* dumb. One of the most important things about training a horse is that you have to be smarter than he is. You have to make sure that you understand what you are trying to teach him.

You really have to watch how horses react to conditioning. Trailering a horse is an experience that is rife with opportunities for conditioning results that you may not be expecting. For instance, your horse seems reluctant to load in the trailer. You come up behind him and hit him with a whip. He loads (or not). The next time, he's worse, so you hit him again. It is not at all inconceivable that your horse will begin to associate loading into a horse trailer with being hit (as opposed to associating *not* loading with being hit, as you would hope).

It's pretty easy to overinterpret horse behavior. Horses do what they do for reasons. Horses are not logical or rational, but they are consistent. They firmly believe that because "b" follows "a," "a" caused "b." So it sometimes becomes quite a challenge for the observer (you) to try to figure out what the "a" is that caused the "b" from the horse. Since you are the only one of the two of you who can think, it is your responsibility to try to assess the consequences of your behavior on the horse.

If your horse starts to do something that you don't like, there is most likely a reason for it. Most of the time the reason is quite simple. Some of the time that reason isn't apparent. You will have to observe your horse and think about what is happening to try to figure the reason out. You have to love a sense of mystery to keep horses.

17

Pet Peeves

Finally, it's time to bring up a few health myths that have no basis in good medicine (or reality, for that matter). These persist because of the unconscious but determined efforts of horse professionals and nonprofessionals alike. Some day, hopefully, they will fade away.

Horses very rarely get sore backs because their kidneys hurt. People do. When a person has a kidney stone, one of the most common signs is excruciating lower back pain. The kidneys generally work just great in horses, and kidney stones are very uncommon. When kidney problems do occur in horses, signs such as decreased appetite, poor performance or hind limb lameness may be seen, and these signs are much more common than back pain. The incidence of kidney stones in horses is terribly (and fortunately) rare.[1]

Mares do not get sore backs because of ovarian cysts. Women get ovarian cysts. So do cattle. Horses do not. The cystic ovary that is seen in other species does not occur in horses.[2] Mares can develop a variety of ovarian abnormalities but not cystic ovaries. Mares can have abnormalities of breeding follicles (the structure on the ovaries from which the egg is produced). These occur most commonly at the beginning or end of the breeding cycle, when mares are in transition from a normal cycle to their normal period of inactivity. Abnormalities of ovarian follicles are not associated with back pain and poor performance, however.

If you think your horse has a sore back, have it evaluated by a professional. There is a proper method for obtaining a diagnosis of back problems.[3] Just because a horse bends when you push on his back does not mean that his back hurts. Back soreness may occur from a poorly fitting saddle.[4] It also occurs commonly in association with lameness of the back legs. Don't worry so much about kidneys and ovaries in sore-backed horses.

Foals do not need shots when they are born. They get their immunity (antibodies) from the colostrum (first milk) of the mare. It is important that the foals drink vigorously in the first few hours of life. The high levels of immunity that a foal gets from his mother last two to three months. These levels of colostral antibody actually prevent a horse from responding to vaccinations such as tetanus toxoid and eliminate the need for a tetanus antitoxin injection. For some reason, some healthy foals are also given a shot of penicillin (just in case?) and sometimes a shot of vitamins, too.[5] At least vitamins are harmless. Stop poking babies.

What is important with newborns is to make sure that they get adequate colostrum. There are a variety of blood tests available to check that they have absorbed enough colostrum. If a foal does not absorb adequate colostrum, he is at high risk for developing a variety of neonatal diseases.[5] If this failure to absorb antibodies is recognized early, foals can be treated to help prevent the serious diseases that can occur in unprotected babies.

Newborn babies do not always need an enema. (Why do people insist on tormenting their new babies?) When babies are born, their intestines have a plug in them called the meconium. This is a dark, hard material that is a mixture of intestinal secretions and fluid from the amnion. Foals will ordinarily just push it on out, sometimes with a little straining. In some new foals the meconium can be retained and require treatment for its removal, but this is rare.[5]

Giving your horse a gallon of mineral oil prior to shipping him doesn't keep him from colicking during the ride. There is nothing that has been proven to prevent a colic. If you give your horse mineral oil, however, it will guarantee you a mess in the trailer.

There is no "best" way to take horses over long distances. While some haulers prefer to stop periodically and get the horse out of the trailer so that he can rest or relax (sometimes even scheduling stops at horse motels along the way), many others prefer to load the horse on the trailer and go straight through to their destination (making sure that the horse has adequate food and water, of course). There's absolutely no evidence to indicate that one way is better than another, but if you haul straight through, you'll get to your destination faster.

There is a condition of horses called shipping fever (or pleuropneumonia, in medical terms). This most commonly occurs after transport, though, of course, not all horses that have been shipped develop it. Shipping fever is a disease of the lungs and the chest cavity caused by bacteria. It is a serious condition. The stress of transport is thought to have something to do with the development of the disease.

Nothing has been shown to prevent shipping fever. Practices such as giving a horse a shot of antibiotics prior to transport, while the motives are understandable, have not been demonstrated to be effective in preventing the condition. Sometimes transported horses are given nonsteroidal anti-inflammatory drugs to help decrease the stress. This has not been shown to be helpful in preventing shipping fever either. In fact, the use of such drugs may suppress the early clinical signs of fever and could conceivably allow the condition to progress before treatment is initiated.[6]

If you ship your horse, make sure that you have a nice trailer (that is driven sensibly) and plenty of feed and water available. If you'd like to put on bandages to protect your horse's legs, why not? And keep your fingers crossed.

Horses don't grow long coats of hair because it gets cold. The growth of hair (and shedding) is primarily stimulated by the change in the length of the day.[7] Hair growth is thought to be controlled by the pineal gland, a small gland at the base of the brain. Horses in warm climates will still grow a "winter" hair coat as the days get shorter.

Horses don't need blankets to stay warm in the winter, even if they have been body clipped, except possibly in the coldest climates. Horses have a hard time staying cool, but they have no trouble at all keeping body heat. This is because of the biogeometry of the horse.

Assume that all animals are spheres (albeit with legs attached). The smaller the sphere, the greater the proportion of its surface is exposed when compared to a larger sphere. The more the surface of something that is exposed, the more area that is available for heat loss. Or, to put it the other way, the larger the animal (the sphere), the less surface is exposed proportional to its size and the harder it is for it to get rid of heat.

Horses have a terrible time staying cool, especially in hot weather. That's one of the reasons why they sweat so much. But ever notice how frisky horses get when it's cold? They must think it's just great to be actually comfortable. Blankets do keep the coats clean and they may have some use if it's very cold and you clipped off all of your horse's hair coat so that he will dry off more quickly or so that he will look better at horse shows. Mostly, blankets make the horse *owners* feel better.

Male foals don't come from the right ovary nor do female foals come from the left ovary. Nor vice versa.

You don't always have to put horses to sleep when they break their legs. There are a lot of factors involved in what happens to a horse after he breaks his leg.

First, a lot depends on what bone is broken. Horses almost never have to be put to sleep when they break the bone of the foot, for example. But a fracture of the hip in an adult horse may be irreparable, for no other reason than it is virtually impossible to get to.

Second, much depends on the extent of the injury. While racing, so much stress can be applied to the horse's leg that, when it breaks, it can almost literally explode, destroying all of the tissue in the leg in the process. In these unfortunate cases, there is nothing left to repair. The horse is put to sleep for humane reasons.

Third, the future of the horse must be taken into consideration. Unfortunately, after some fractures have healed there will be some degree of lameness as a result. This is a particular problem with fractures of a joint. When a bone fractures into a joint, it may be impossible to return the joint surface to normal. Consequently, the resulting repaired surface can frequently and unavoidably begin a progression to degenerative arthritis.

While it may be fine to have a broodmare or a valuable stallion limp around a bit with a repaired fracture, the same result may not at all be desirable in a gelding that is supposed to jump fences. Unless the owner of the gelding wants to have (and pay for) a horse that can only be looked at and brushed, sometimes euthanasia of the horse is a reasonable, though tragic, result of a fracture.

Horse bones can be exceedingly difficult to repair. The large bones of the upper legs, for instance, are difficult to approach surgically. To get to them, a great deal of tissue has to be cut through (and traumatized), leading to more pain for the horse and opening up the leg to the potential for infection. Sometimes, even the best repairs go sour.

As a final factor and complication, horses are terrible orthopedic patients. They are big animals, and a fractured leg has to bear a lot of weight. Not only that, but the fractured leg has to begin to bear that weight *immediately* after the repair has been performed. Horses won't lie down in bed and watch television until the bone heals (and they can't use crutches). Sometimes the implants that are used to hold the bone together aren't even strong enough to take the pressure of the horse's weight. A single awkward or improper step can bend a metal bone plate just as if it were a paper clip and destroy several hours of difficult surgery (and the horse). If a horse will not bear weight on the fractured leg after it has been repaired, problems such as laminitis in the other leg can develop, because the horse cannot bear all of his weight on just one leg.

Some fractures in horses can be repaired and some can't. There are a lot of things to consider. But you don't have to put them all to sleep.

Veterinarians don't usually shoot horses to put them to sleep. (It can be done, and if done properly, it is quick and humane.) Veterinarians usually use an overdose of a barbiturate, injected intravenously. The horses go very quickly to sleep (literally) and do not wake up.

You can't catch your horse's cold. Viruses and bacteria that make horses sick cannot make people sick. You *can* get ringworm, a fungal skin infection, from them.

There's no good reason to keep a stallion unless you run a breeding operation. Stallions can be unpredictable and dangerous. A castrated horse is more docile, more predictable, easier to handle and safer to be around than a stallion. People seem to have this romantic notion of the powerful stallion. Give it up.

When horses are castrated, their testicles are removed. The testicles produce the male hormone testosterone, which makes stallions such a pain. There is no other tissue in the horse's body that makes testosterone.

People worry that their horses will be proud cut, that is, if the testicles aren't cut off far enough away from the testicle, the new gelding will still act like a stallion. This isn't possible. As mentioned above, the testicle is the only structure that makes testosterone, and if it's gone there is no other source of this hormone—no matter how "close" to the testicle the cut was made. If the testicle is completely removed and the gelding still acts like an idiot, it's his personality, not the fault of the surgery.

Castrate your horse early, before he's a yearling. This does not stunt a horse's growth, nor does it make him weaker than he might have been otherwise. There's less trauma and swelling associated with the surgery when you castrate early.

Just because your horse is sick, don't feel compelled to give him *something*. If your horse has a colic, don't use whiskey, baking soda, frozen apple juice, turpentine, castor oil or anything else that's weird. Don't use products containing atropine (some are available) to treat colic. Atropine can stop the intestines from moving.[8] This can cause the death of the horse all by itself.

If you have a question about what to do for your horse's health, call your *veterinarian* to ask for advice.

Epilogue

It is amazing that horses have survived their owners, what with all the legend and lore about what must be done to them. Most things involving the care of a horse are pretty simple and make sense. If something doesn't make sense to you, then it's probably not right. Beware of anyone who says that you have to take care of your horse in a certain fashion, or else something else bad will happen. Undoubtedly, not everyone does things the same way, and assuredly not everyone has problems because of the differences.

If you do have health questions, call your veterinarian. If your questions aren't answered to your satisfaction, call a veterinarian with lots of training. Universities and referral hospitals are stuffed with veterinarians who have suffered through many years of specialized training and who would be only too happy to answer your specific questions. Be curious and get your questions answered; after all, your horse is depending on you to take care of him.

Your friends and neighbors are undoubtedly good people. However, they are also fervent keepers of the myths. They are not health professionals; nor are farriers, "chiropractors" or "dentists."

When someone tells you a story that doesn't ring true about your horse's health, don't anger them by telling them that they are wrong. Give them a copy of this book.

Notes

CHAPTER ONE

1. N. A. White, *The Equine Acute Abdomen* (Philadelphia: Lea and Febiger, 1990), 115–16.
2. M. J. Kluger, "The Evolution and Adaptive Value of Fever," *Am. Sci.* 66, no. 1 (1978): 38–43.
3. M. J. Kluger, "Fever and Survival," *Science* 188, no. 4184 (1975): 66–68.
4. M. Banet, "Fever in Mammals: Is It Beneficial?" *Yale J. Bio. Med.* 59, no. 2 (1986): 117–24.
5. M. Kluger, "Is Fever Beneficial?" *Yale J. Bio. Med.* 59, no. 2 (1986): 89–95.
6. C. M. Blatteis, "Fever: Is It Beneficial?" *Yale J. Bio. Med.* 59, no. 2 (1986): 107–16.
7. G. W. Duff, "Is Fever Beneficial to the Host: A Clinical Perspective," *Yale J. Bio. Med.* 59, no. 2 (1986): 125–30.
8. R. Hellon et al., "Mechanisms of Fever," in *Thermoregulation: Pathology, Pharmacology and Therapy* (New York: Pergamon Press, 1991), 42–45.
9. M. Banet, "Fever and Survival in the Rat. Metabolic vs. Temperature Response," *Experientia* 37 (1981): 1302–04.
10. M. J. Kluger, "Temperature Regulation, Fever and Disease," in *International Review of Physiology: Environmental Physiology III*, vol. 20, ed. D. Robertshaw (Baltimore: University Park Press, 1979), 209–51.
11. White, *Equine Acute Abdomen*, 116–24.
12. The packed cell volume is obtained by taking the blood, putting it in a tube and spinning it down in a centrifuge. When a tube of fluid is rapidly spun in a circle, the heavy stuff gets pushed down to the end of the tube on the outer edge of the circle. In the blood, the cells are the heavy stuff. Therefore, when blood gets spun in a centrifuge, all of the cells (red and white) pack down (hence the name) into the end of the spinning tube. The length of the band of cells in the tube is divided by the overall length of the column of fluid in the tube. The resulting number is the packed cell volume measurement. This measurement is then compared with a laboratory list of normals.
13. M. M. Henry, "Diagnostic Approach to Anemia," in *Current Therapy in Equine Medicine III*, ed. N. E. Robinson (Philadelphia: W. B. Saunders, 1992), 487–92.
14. O. W. Schalm, *Manual of Equine Hematology* (Santa Barbara, CA: Veterinary Practice Publishing Co., 1984), 5–10.

15. M. M. Henry, "Anemia Due to Inadequate Erythropoesis," in *Current Therapy III*, 494–95.

16. T. A. Turner, "Thermography as an Aid to Clinical Lameness Evaluation," *Vet. Clin. NA Eq. Prac.* 7, no. 2 (1991): 311–18.

17. T. S. Stashak, *Adams' Lameness in Horses*, 4th ed. (Philadelphia: Lea and Febiger, 1987), 134–50.

18. W. B. Schmotzer and K. I. Timm, "Local Anesthetic Techniques for Diagnosis of Lameness," *Vet. Clin. NA Eq. Prac.* 6, no. 3 (1990): 705–28.

19. V. B. Reef, "Ultrasonic Diagnosis of Tendon and Ligament Disease," in *Current Practice in Equine Surgery*, ed. N. A. White and J. N. Moore (Philadelphia: J. B. Lippincott, 1990), 425–35.

20. V. B. Reef, "Advances in Diagnostic Ultrasonography," *Vet. Clin. NA Eq. Prac.* 7, no. 2 (1991): 451–66.

21. R. R. Steckel, "The Role of Scintigraphy in the Lameness Evaluation," *Vet. Clin. NA Eq. Prac.* 7, no. 2 (1991): 207–39.

CHAPTER TWO

1. *Dorland's Illustrated Medical Dictionary*, 25th ed. (Philadelphia: W. B. Saunders Co., 1974).

2. J. V. Hurley, "Inflammation," in *Edema*, ed. N. C. Staub and A. E. Taylor (New York: Raven Press, 1984), 463–88.

3. T. S. Stashak, *Adams' Lameness in Horses*, 4th ed. (Philadelphia: Lea and Febiger, 1987), 840.

4. T. S. Stashak, *Equine Wound Management* (Philadelphia: Lea and Febiger, 1991), 29.

5. D. Richardson, "Degenerative Joint Disease," in *Current Therapy in Equine Medicine III*, ed. N. E. Robinson (Philadelphia: W. B. Saunders, 1992), 137–40.

6. L. Branlage, "Medical Treatment of Tendinitis," in *Current Therapy III*, 146–49.

7. S. L. Fubini, "Intestinal Adhesions," in *Current Practice of Equine Surgery*, ed. N. A. White and J. N. Moore (Philadelphia: J. B. Lippincott, 1990), 382–84.

8. D. W. Richardson, "Medical Treatment of Degenerative Joint Disease," in *Equine Medicine and Surgery*, 4th ed., ed. P. T. Colahan et al. (Goleta, CA: American Veterinary Publications, 1991), 1258.

9. A. Vachon and C. W. McIlwraith, "Articular Cartilage Healing: Current Concepts," in *Current Practice of Equine Surgery*, 544.

10. J. H. Stevenson et al., "Functional, Mechanical and Biochemical Assessment of Ultrasound Therapy on Tendon Healing in the Chicken Toe," *Plast. and Reconstr. Surg.* 77 (1986): 965–72.

11. T. A. Turner, K. Wolfsdorf and J. Jourdenais, "Effects of Heat, Cold, Biomagnets and Ultrasound on Skin Circulation in the Horse," *Proc. 37th AAEP* (1991): 249–57.

12. A. J. Kaneps et al., "Laser Therapy in the Horse: Histopathologic Response," *A. J. Vet. Res.* 45, no. 3 (1984): 581–82.

13. M. A. Collier et al., "Electrostimulation of Bone Production in the Horse," *Proc. 27th AAEP* (1981): 71–89.

14. D. V. Flynn, "Enhancement of Osteogenesis by Electrostimulation—Non-invasive Technique," *Proc. 27th AAEP* (1981): 91.
15. Stashek, *Adams' Lameness*, 857.
16. H. L. Barnum, *The American Farrier* (1882).
17. I. A. Silver and P. D. Rosedale, "A Clinical and Experimental Study of Tendon Injury, Healing and Treatment in the Horse," *Eq. Vet. J.*, suppl. 1 (July 1983): 1–39.
18. S. L. Willoughby, "Equine Chiropractic Care," *Proc. 39th AAEP* (1993): 31, 32.
19. International Veterinary Chiropractic Association, P.O. Box 249, Port Byron, IL 61275, (309) 523–3995.
20. B. B. Martin and A. M. Klide, "Acupuncture for the Treatment of Chronic Back Pain in 200 Horses," *Proc. 37th AAEP* (1991): 593–601.
21. Stashak, *Adams' Lameness*, 866.
22. Stashak, *Adams' Lameness*, 857.
23. Stashak, *Adams' Lameness*, 858–62.

CHAPTER THREE

1. R. D. Walker, "Antimicrobial Chemotherapy," in *Current Therapy in Equine Medicine III*, ed. N. E. Robinson (Philadelphia: W. B. Saunders, 1992), 12.
2. S. A. May, "Anti-inflammatory Agents," in *Current Therapy III*, 14–18.
3. N. H. Booth and L. E. McDonald, *Veterinary Pharmacology and Therapeutics*, 6th ed. (Ames: Iowa State University Press, 1988), 38–69.
4. A. J. Nixon, "Intra-articular Medication," in *Current Therapy III*, 127–28.
5. S. Chunekamrai et al., "Changes in Articular Cartilage after Intra-articular Injection of Methylprednisolone Acetate in Horses," *A.J. Vet. Res.* 50 (1989): 1733–41.
6. C. G. Van Arman, D. Armstrong and D. H. Kim, "Antipyretics," in *Thermoregulation: Pathology, Pharmacology and Therapy*, ed. E. Shonbaum and P. Lomax (New York: Pergamon Press, 1991), 55–104.
7. M. Kalpravidh, "Effects of Butorphanol, Flunixin, Levorphanol, Morphine and Xylazine in Ponies," *A.J. Vet. Res.* 45 (1984): 217–23.
8. W. Jochle et al., "Comparison of Detomodine, Butorphanol, Flunixin Meglumine and Xylazine in Clinical Cases of Equine Colic," *Eq. Vet. J.*, suppl. 7 (1989): 111–16.
9. E. S. Clark, "Pharmacologic Management of Colic," in *Current Therapy III*, 201–206.
10. G. M. Baxter, "Laminitis," in *Current Therapy III*, 154–60.
11. D. H. Snow, "Phenylbutazone Toxicity," in *Current Therapy in Equine Medicine II*, ed. N. E. Robinson (Philadelphia: W. B. Saunders, 1987), 118–19.
12. R. M. Bednarski, "Chemical Restraint of the Standing Horse," in *Current Therapy III*, 22–25.
13. K. A. Houpt, "Stable Vices and Trailer Problems," *Vet. Clin. NA Eq. Prac.* 2, no. 3 (1986): 630.
14. M. J. Reeves et al., "Failure to Demonstrate Reperfusion Injury Following Ischemia of the Equine Large Colon Using Dimethyl Sulfoxide," *Eq. Vet. J.* 22 (1990): 122–26.
15. J. E. Sojka et al., "Dimethyl Sulfoxide Update—New Applications and Dosing Methods," in *Proc. 36th AAEP* (1990): 683–90.

Chapter Four

1. *Nutrient Requirements of Horses*, 5th rev. ed. (Washington, DC: National Academy Press: 1989), 37.
2. *Nutrient Requirements*, 3–4.
3. P. L. Hambleton et al., "Dietary Fat and Exercise Conditioning Effect on Metabolic Parameters in the Horse," *J. An. Sci.* 51 (1980): 1330.
4. S. E. Duren et al., "Effect of Dietary Fat on Blood Parameters in Exercised Thoroughbred Horses," in *Equine Exercise Physiology II*, ed. J. R. Gillespie and N. E. Robinson (Davis, CA: ICEEP Publications, 1987), 674–84.
5. H. L. Hintz et al., "Effects of Protein Level on Endurance Horses," *Proc. 72nd Ann. Meet. Am. Soc. An. Sci.* (1980): 202.
6. S. L. Ralston, "Nutritional Management of Horses Competing in 160 Km Races," *Cornell Vet.* 78 (1988): 53.
7. *Dorland's Illustrated Medical Dictionary*, 25th ed. (Philadelphia: W. B. Saunders, 1974).
8. *Nutrient Requirements*, 210.
9. D. C. Church and W. G. Pond, *Basic Animal Nutrition and Feeding* (Corvallis, OR: D. C. Church, 1976), 9.

Chapter Five

1. *Nutrient Requirements of Horses*, 5th rev. ed. (Washington, DC: National Academy Press, 1989), 37.
2. The following table of individual condition scores is taken from *Nutrient Requirements of Horses* and adapted from D. R. Henneke, "Relationship between Condition Score, Physical Measurement and Body Fat Percentage in Mares," *Eq. Vet. J.* 15 (1983): 371.

Score	Description
1 (Poor)	Extremely emaciated; spinous processes, ribs, tailhead, tuber coxae and ischii project prominently; bone structure of withers, shoulders and neck easily noticeable; no fatty tissue can be felt.
2 (Very thin)	Emaciated; slight fat covering over base of spinous processes; transverse spinous processes cannot be felt; vertebrae feel rounded; spinous processes, ribs, tailhead, tuber coxae and ischii prominent; withers, shoulders and neck structures are faintly discernible.
3 (Thin)	Fat buildup about halfway on spinous process; transverse spinous process cannot be felt; slight fat cover over ribs; spinous processes easily felt; tailhead prominent but individual vertebrae cannot be identified visually; tuber coxae rounded but easily seen; tuber ischii not apparent; withers, neck and shoulder accentuated.
4 (Moderately thin)	Slight ridge along back; faint outline of ribs discernible; tailhead prominence depends on conformation, fat can be felt around it; tuber coxae not discernible; withers, shoulders and neck not obviously thin.

5 (Moderate)   Back is flat (no crease or ridge); ribs not visually distinguishable but easily felt; fat around tailhead beginning to feel spongy; withers appear rounded over spinous processes; shoulders and neck blend smoothly into body.

6 (Moder-   May have slight crease down back; fat over ribs is spongy; fat around
ately fleshy)   tailhead soft; fat beginning to be deposited along the side of withers, behind shoulders and along neck.

7 (Fleshy)   May have crease down back; individual ribs can be felt, but noticeable filling between ribs with fat; fat around tailhead soft; fat deposited along withers, behind shoulders and along neck.

8 (Fat)   Crease down back; difficult to feel ribs; fat around tailhead very soft; area along withers filled with fat; area behind shoulders filled with fat; noticeable thickening of neck; fat deposited along inner thighs.

9 (Extremely   Obvious crease down back; patchy fat over ribs; bulging fat around
fat)   tailhead, along withers, behind shoulders and along neck; fat along inner thighs may rub together; flank filled with fat.

3. L. D. Lewis, Animal Nutrition Notes, Colorado State University, 1981.
4. *Nutrient Requirements*, 7, 39–40.
5. D. L. Frape, "Dietary Requirements and Athletic Performance of Horses," *Eq. Vet. J.* 2, no. 3 (1988): 163–72.
6. *Nutrition Requirements*, 37.
7. M. J. Glade, "Nutrition for the Equine Athlete," in *Equine Sports Medicine*, ed. W. E. Jones (Philadelphia: Lea and Febiger, 1989), 19–30.
8. H. F. Hintz, "Nutritional Requirements of the Exercising Horse—A Review," in *Equine Exercise Physiology, Proc. 1st Int. Conf.*, ed. D. H. Snow, S. G. B. Persson and R. J. Rose (Cambridge, England: Granta Editions, 1982), 275–90.
9. H. F. Hintz, *Horse Nutrition: A Practical Guide* (New York: Arco Publishing, 1982).
10. N. E. Lopez, J. P. Baker and S. G. Jackson, "Effect of Cutting and Vacuum Cleaning on the Digestibility of Oats by Horses," *J. Eq. Vet. Sci.* 8 (1988): 375–77.
11. D. L. Costill, "Carbohydrate Nutrition Before, During and After Exercise," *Fed. Pro.* 44 (1985): 364–68.
12. M. Gleeson, R. J. Maughan and P. L. Greenhaff, "Effects of Pre-Exercise Feeding of Glycerol or Glucose on Metabolism and Endurance Performance in Man," *Proc. Nutr. Soc.* 45 (1986): 127A.
13. H. F. Hintz, "Some Myths About Equine Nutrition," *Comp. Cont. Ed.* 12, no. 1 (1990): 79–81, 89.
14. H. Meyer et al., "Investigation of Sodium Deficiencies in Horses," in *Proc. 8th Eq. Nutr. and Physiol. Symposium* (Lexington, KY, 1983): 11.
15. R. D. Goodrich, D. E. Pamp and J. C. Merske, "Free Choice Minerals," *Proc. Minnesota Nutr. Conf.* (1977): 171–77.
16. H. F. Hintz, "Equine Nutrition" (paper presented at Annual Conference for Veterinarians, Colorado State University, 1977).

17. H. F. Schryver and H. F. Hintz, "Recent Developments in Equine Nutrition," *An. Nut. and Health* 4 (1975): 6–10.

18. S. L. Ralston, "Feeding Behavior," *Vet. Clin. NA Eq. Prac.* 2, no. 3 (1986): 611.

19. H. F. Schryver et al., "The Voluntary Intake of Calcium by Horses and Ponies," *J. Eq. Med. Surg.* 2 (1978): 337.

20. S. L. Ralston, "Feeding Behavior," 617.

21. G. P. Carlson, P. O. Ocen and D. Harrold, "Clinicopathological Alterations in Normal and Exhausted Endurance Horses," *Theriogenology* 6 (1976): 93–104.

22. G. P. Carlson, "Thermoregulation and Fluid Balance in the Exercising Horse," in *Equine Exercise Physiology*, 291–309.

23. G. P. Carlson, "The Exhausted Horse Syndrome," in *Current Therapy in Equine Medicine II*, ed. N. E. Robinson (Philadelphia: W. B. Saunders, 1987), 482–85.

24. G. P. Carlson, "Synchronous Diaphragmatic Flutter," in *Current Therapy II*, 485–86.

25. S. L. Ralston, "Feeding Behavior," 616.

CHAPTER SIX

1. *Nutrient Requirements of Horses*, 5th rev. ed. (Washington, DC: National Academy Press, 1989).

2. W. L. Beard and D. A. Knight, "Developmental Orthopedic Disease," in *Current Therapy in Equine Medicine III*, ed. N. E. Robinson (Philadelphia: W. B. Saunders, 1992), 105–109.

3. M. A. Williams, "Risk Factors Associated with Developmental Orthopedic Disease," in *Current Therapy III*, 462–65.

4. D. S. Kronfeld, T. N. Meacham and S. Donoghue, "Dietary Aspects of Developmental Orthopedic Disease in Young Horses," *Vet. Clin. NA Eq. Prac.* 6, no. 2 (1990): 451–65.

5. D. A. Knight et al., "The Effects of Copper Supplementation on the Prevalence of Cartilage Lesions in Foals," *Eq. Vet. J.* 22, no. 6 (1990): 426–32.

6. L. R. Bramlage, "Investigation of Farm Wide Incidence of Bone Formation Problems in the Horse," *Proc. 39th AAEP* (1993): 45–48.

7. K. A. Houpt, "Ingestive Behavior," *Vet. Clin. NA Eq. Prac.* 6, no. 2 (1990): 319–37.

8. H. F. Hintz, "Feeding Programs," in *Current Therapy in Equine Medicine II*, ed. N. E. Robinson (Philadelphia: W. B. Saunders, 1987), 412–18.

9. M. J. Glade and N. K. Luba, "Serum Triiodothyronine and Thyroxine Concentrations in Weanling Horses Fed Carbohydrate by Direct Gastric Infusion," *Am. J. Vet. Res.* 48 (1987): 578.

10. M. J. Glade and T. H. Belling, Jr., "Growth Plate Cartilage Metabolism, Morphology and Biochemical Composition in Over- and Underfed Horses," *Growth* (1984): 473.

11. M. J. Glade and T. J. Reimers, "Effects of Dietary Energy Supply on Serum Thyroxine, Triiodothyronine and Insulin Concentrations in Young Horses," *J. Endocr.* 104 (1985): 93.

12. K. N. Thompson, S. J. Jackson and J. R. Rooney, "The Effect of Above Average Weight Gains on the Incidence of Radiographic Bone Aberrations and Epiphysitis in Growing Horses," *Proc. 20th Eq. Nutr. Physiol. Soc.* (Fort Collins, CO, 1987): 5.

13. B, D Soott et al., "Growth and Feed Utilization by Yearling Horses Fed Added Dietary Fat," *Proc. 20th Eq. Nutr.* 101–106.
14. H. F. Schryver et al., "Growth and Calcium Metabolism in Horses Fed Varying Levels of Protein," *Eq. Vet. J.* 19 (1987): 280.
15. E. A. Ott and R. L. Asquith, "Influence of Level of Feeding and Nutrient Content of the Concentrate on Growth and Development of Yearling Horses," *J. An. Sci.* 62 (1986): 290.
16. H. F. Hintz, "Factors Which Influence Developmental Orthopedic Disease," *Proc. 33rd AAEP Eq. Prac.* (1987): 159–62.
17. D. S. Kronfeld and S. Donoghue, "Metabolic Convergence in Developmental Orthopedic Disease," *Proc. 33rd AAEP* (1987): 195–202.
18. H. F. Hintz, "Some Myths About Equine Nutrition," *Comp. Cont. Ed.* 12, no. 1 (1990): 79–81, 89.
19. S. Donoghue, T. N. Meacham and D. S. Kronfeld, "A Conceptual Approach to Optimal Nutrition of the Brood Mare," *Vet. Clin. NA Eq. Prac.* 6, no. 2 (1990): 373–91.
20. S. L. Ralston, C. F. Nockels and E. L. Squires, "Hematologic, Metabolic and Digestive Changes in Aged Horses," *Proc. 10th Eq. Nutr.:* 545.
21. S. L. Ralston, "Digestion in the Aged Horse," *J. Eq. Vet. Sci.* (1989): 203–205.
22. S. L. Ralston, "Clinical Nutrition of Adult Horses," *Vet. Clin. NA Eq. Prac.* 6, no. 2 (1990): 339–54.

Chapter Seven

1. *Dorland's Illustrated Medical Dictionary*, 25th ed. (Philadelphia: W. B. Saunders, 1974).
2. I. R. Tizard, *An Introduction to Veterinary Immunology* (Philadelphia: W. B. Saunders, 1977).
3. H. Gerber, "Clinical Features, Sequelae and Epidemiology of Equine Influenza," in *Equine Infectious Disease II*, ed. J. T. Bryans and H. Gerber (New York: Karger, 1969), 63–80.
4. W. D. Wilson, "Equine Influenza," *Vet. Clin. NA Eq. Prac.* 9, no. 2 (1993): 257–82.
5. J. T. Mumford et al., "Studies with Inactivated Equine Influenza Vaccine. 2. Protection Against Experimental Infection with Influenza Virus A/Equine Newmarket/79 (H3N8). *J. Hyg. Camb.* 90 (1983): 385–95.
6. D. G. Powell et al., "Field Observations on Influenza Vaccination Among Horses in Britain, 1971–1976," *Intl. Symp. on Influenza Immunology (II) Devel. Biol. Stand.* 39 (1977): 347–52.
7. J. M. Wood et al., "Studies with Inactivated Equine Influenza Vaccine. 1. Serological Responses of Ponies to Graded Doses of Vaccine," *J. Hyg. Camb.* 90 (1982): 371–84.
8. E. N. Ostlund, "The Equine Herpesviruses," *Vet. Clin. NA Eq. Prac.* 9, no. 2 (1993): 283–94.
9. A. C. Pickles, "Vaccination of Mares Against Equine Herpesvirus-1," *Vet. Rec.*, letter, Feb. 22, 1992: 167.
10. B. C. Jansen and P. C. Knoetze, "The Immune Response of Horses to Tetanus Toxoid," *Onderstespoort J. Vet. Res.* 46 (1979): 211.
11. R. McConnico, "Tetanus," in *Current Therapy in Equine Medicine III*, ed. N. E. Robinson (Philadelphia: W. B. Saunders, 1992), 540–41.

12. J. Johnston, "Tetanus," in *Current Therapy in Equine Medicine II*, ed. N. E. Robinson (Philadelphia: W. B. Saunders, 1987), 370–73.
13. A. M. Koterba, "Diagnosis and Management of the Normal and Abnormal Neonatal Foal: General Considerations," in *Equine Clinical Neonatology*, ed. A. M. Koterba, W. H. Drumond and P. C. Kosch (Philadelphia: Lea and Febiger, 1990), 5–6.
14. J. J. Bertone, "Togaviral Encephalitides: Alphavirus (Eastern and Western) Equine Encephalitis," in *Current Therapy III*, 547–50.
15. J. Palmer, "Potomac Horse Fever," *Vet. Clin. NA Eq. Prac.* 9, no. 2 (1993): 399–410.
16. J. E. Sessions and J. Dawson, "Product Evaluation: Maryland Field Evaluation of the Potomac Horse Fever Vaccine," *Eq. Prac.* 10 (1988): 7.
17. M. Ristic, C. J. Holland and T. E. Goetz, "Evaluation of a Vaccine for Equine Monocytic Ehrlichiosis," *Proc. Sym. Potomac Horse Fever* (Louisville, KY, 1988): 89.
18. S. L. Green, "Equine Rabies," *Vet. Clin. NA Eq. Prac.* 9, no. 2 (1993): 337–47.
19. P. A. Pintchuk, "Botulism," in *Current Therapy III*, 542–44.
20. P. J. Timoney and W. H. McCollum, "Equine Viral Arteritis," *Vet. Clin. NA Eq. Prac.* 9, no. 2 (1993): 295–309.
21. P. J. Timoney et al., "Demonstration of the Carrier State in Naturally Acquired Equine Arteritis Virus Infections in the Stallion," *Res. Vet. Sci.* 41 (1986): 279.
22. P. J. Timoney and W. H. McCollum, "Equine Viral Arteritis. Current Clinical and Economic Significance," *Proc. 36th AAEP* (1990): 403.

CHAPTER EIGHT

1. "Parasitology," *Vet. Clin. NA Eq. Prac.* 2, no. 2 (1986).
2. J. H. Drudge and E. T. Lyons, "Large Strongyles: Recent Advances," *Vet. Clin. NA Eq. Prac.* 2, no. 2 (1986): 263–80.
3. R. P. Hackett, "Ileocecal Intussusception," in *Current Practice of Equine Surgery*, ed. N. A. White and J. N. Moore (Philadelphia: J. B. Lippincott, 1990), 328.
4. J. A. DiPietro and K. S. Todd, "Anthelmintics Used in Treatment of Parasitic Infection of Horses," *Vet. Clin. NA Eq. Prac.* 3, no. 1 (1987): 1–14.
5. J. A. DiPietro, "Internal Parasite Control Programs," *Current Therapy in Equine Medicine III*, ed. N. E. Robinson (Philadelphia: W. B. Saunders, 1992), 51–55.
6. C. Uhlinger and M. Kristula, "A Field Evaluation of Three Methods of Administration of Anthelmintics to Horses," *Eq. Vet. J.* 24, no. 6 (1992): 487–89.
7. W. D. Wilson, "Foal Pneumonia," in *Current Therapy III*, 466–73.
8. H. M. Clayton, "Ascarids: Recent Advances," *Vet. Clin. NA Eq. Prac.* 2, no. 2 (1986): 313–28.
9. R. P. Herd, "Pasture Hygiene: A Nonchemical Approach to Equine Endoparasite Control," *Mod. Vet. Prac.* 67 (1986): 36–38.
10. R. P. Herd, "Epidemiology and Control of Parasites in Northern Temperate Regions," *Vet. Clin. NA Eq. Prac.* 2, no. 2 (1986): 337–55.
11. R. P. Herd, "Monitoring Control Programs," in *Current Therapy in Equine Medicine II*, ed. N. E. Robinson (Philadelphia: W. B. Saunders, 1987), 336–37.
12. T. M. Craig and C. H. Courtney, "Epidemiology and Control of Parasites in Warm Climates," *Vet. Clin. NA Eq. Prac.* 2, no. 2 (1986): 362.

CHAPTER NINE

1. C. Uhlinger, "Common Abnormalities of the Premolars and Molars," *Proc. 37th AAEP* (1991): 123–28.
2. W. L. Scrutchfield, "Incisors and Canines," *Proc. 37th AAEP* (1991): 117–22.
3. G. J. Baker, "Dental Morphology, Function and Pathology," *Proc. 37th AAEP* (1991): 83–94.
4. J. Richardson, "Aging the Horse: A Fresh View of an Old Concept," *Proc. 33rd British Eq. Vet. Assn.* (1994): 86.
5. K. J. Easley, "Recognition and Management of the Diseased Equine Tooth," *Proc. 37th AAEP* (1991): 129–40.

CHAPTER TEN

1. *Dorland's Illustrated Medical Dictionary*, 25th ed. (Philadelphia: W. B. Saunders, 1974).
2. N. A. White, "Intensive Care, Monitoring and Complications of Acute Abdominal Disease," in *The Equine Acute Abdomen*, ed. N. A. White (Philadelphia: Lea and Febiger, 1990), 309–36.
3. A. T. Fisher, "Diagnostic and Prognostic Procedures for Equine Colic Surgery," *Vet. Clin. NA Eq. Prac.* 5, no. 2 (1989): 335–50.
4. N. A. White, "Examination and Diagnosis of the Acute Abdomen," in *Equine Acute Abdomen*, 102–42.
5. N. A. White and T. D. Byars, "Analgesia," in *Equine Acute Abdomen*, 154.
6. A. Wagner. ["Statistics on Equine Colic and Relationships to Climatic Conditions"] (inaugural diss., Fachbereich Veterinarmedizin, Freie Universitat, Berlin, Germany, 1990).
7. M. Reeves, "Risk and Prognostic Factors in Colic," in *Current Therapy in Equine Medicine III*, ed. N. E. Robinson (Philadelphia: W. B. Saunders, 1992), 207.
8. N. A. White, "Epidemiology and Etiology of Colic," in *Equine Acute Abdomen*, 56.
9. S. L. Ralston, "Feeding Behavior," *Vet. Clin. NA Eq. Prac.* 2, no. 3 (1986): 609–22.
10. E. S. Clark, "Intestinal Motility," in *Equine Acute Abdomen*, 39–40.
11. Y. Ruckebusch, "Motor Functions of the Intestine," *Adv. Vet. Sci. Comp. Med.* 25 (1981): 345–69.
12. H. F. Hintz, *Horse Nutrition: A Practical Guide* (New York: Arco Publishing, 1982), 135.
13. H. F. Hintz and J. R. Snyder, "Enterolithiasis," in *Current Therapy III*, 223–25.
14. D. O. Morris, J. N. Moore and S. Ward, "Comparison of Age, Sex, Breed, History and Management in 229 Horses with Colic," *Eq. Vet. J.*, suppl. 7 (June 1989): 129–32.
15. P. Colahan, "Sand Colic," in *Current Therapy in Equine Medicine II*, ed. N. E. Robinson (Philadelphia: W. B. Saunders, 1987), 55–58.
16. E. S. Clark, "Pharmacologic Management of Colic," in *Current Therapy III*, 201–206.
17. P. M. Lish, "Some Pharmacologic Effects of Dioctyl Sodium Sulfosuccinate on the Gastrointestinal Tract of the Rat," *Gastroenterology* 4 (1961): 580.

Chapter Eleven

1. F. G. R. Taylor, "Strangles," in *Current Therapy in Equine Medicine III*, ed. N. E. Robinson (Philadelphia: W. B. Saunders, 1992), 324–26.
2. J. F. Timoney, "Strangles," *Vet. Clin. NA Eq. Prac.* 9, no. 2 (1993): 365–74.
3. A. M. Hoffman et al., "Field Evaluation of a Commercial M Protein Vaccine against *S. equi* Infection in Foals," *Am. J. Vet. Res.* 52 (1991): 52.
4. J. F. Timoney, "*Streptococcus equi*: Current Thinking on Protective Immunity," *Proc. 36th AAEP* (1990): 411.
5. V. B. Reef, "Vasculitis," in *Current Therapy in Equine Medicine II*, ed. N. E. Robinson (Philadelphia: W. B. Saunders, 1987), 312–13.
6. J. T. Bryans and B. O. Moore, "Group C Streptococcal Infections of the Horse," in *Streptococci and Streptococcal Diseases, Recognition, Understanding and Management*, ed. Warmamaker and Matsen (New York: Academic Press, 1972), 329.

Chapter Twelve

1. O. W. Schalm, N. C. Jain and E. J. Carroll, *Veterinary Hematology*, 3rd ed. (Philadelphia: Lea and Febiger, 1975), 291.
2. T. S. Stashak, *Equine Wound Management* (Philadelphia: Lea and Febiger, 1991), 38.
3. W. Lineweaver et al., "Topical Antimicrobial Toxicity," *Arch. Surg.* 120 (1985): 267.
4. A. S. Turner and C. W. McIlwraith, *Techniques in Large Animal Surgery* (Philadelphia: Lea and Febiger, 1982), 98–101.
5. Stashak, *Equine Wound Management*, 22–28.
6. Stashak, *Equine Wound Management*, 11–15.
7. S. F. Swaim, *Surgery of Traumatized Skin: Management and Reconstruction in the Dog and Cat* (Philadelphia: W. B. Saunders, 1980), 83.
8. Stashak, *Equine Wound Management*, 43–44.
9. Stashak, *Equine Wound Management*, 45–48.
10. Stashak, *Equine Wound Management*, 144–49.
11. Stashak, *Equine Wound Management*, 70–88.
12. Stashak, *Equine Wound Management*, 29–32.
13. E. E. Peacock, *Wound Management*, 3rd ed. (Philadelphia: W. B. Saunders, 1984), 158.

Chapter Thirteen

1. W. Moyer, "Clinical Examination of the Equine Foot," *Vet. Clin. NA Eq. Prac.* 5, no. 1 (1989): 29.
2. D. M. Goble, "Medical Evaluation of the Musculoskeletal System and Common Integument Relevant to Purchase," *Vet. Clin. NA Eq. Prac.* 8 no. 2 (1992): 295–301.
3. T. S. Stashak, *Adams' Lameness in Horses*, 4th ed. (Philadelphia: Lea and Febiger, 1987), 357–60.

4. Stashak, *Adams' Lameness*, 844.

5. W. H. Crawford et al., "The Energy Absorption Capacity of Equine Support Bandages: Part 1: Comparison Between Bandages Placed in Various Configurations and Tensions," *Vet. Comp. Orthop. Traum.*, I (1990): 2–9.

6. C. N. Kobluk, "A Kinematic Investigation of the Effect of a Cohesive Elastic Bandage on the Gait of the Exercising Thoroughbred Racehorse," *Proc. 34th AAEP* (1988): 135–48.

7. Stashak, *Adams' Lameness*, 80.

8. Stashak, *Adams' Lameness*, 71.

9. A. Vachon and C. W. McIlwraith, "Articular Cartilage Healing: Current Concepts," in *Current Practice of Equine Surgery*, ed. N. A. White and J. N. Moore (Philadelphia: J. B. Lippincott, 1990), 539–45.

10. G. W. Trotter, "Interphalangeal Degenerative Joint Disease," in *Current Practice of Equine Surgery*, 546–50.

11. T. C. Bohanon, R. K. Schneider and S. W. Weisbrode, "Fusion of the Distal Intertarsal and Tarsometatarsal Joints in the Horse Using Intra-Articular Sodium Moniodoacetate" *Eq. Vet. J.* 23, no. 4 (1991): 289–95.

12. C. W. McIlwraith and A. S. Turner, *Equine Surgery: Advanced Techniques* (Philadelphia: Lea and Febiger, 1987), 185–90.

13. L. R. Bramlage, "Medical Treatment of Tendinitis," in *Current Therapy in Equine Medicine III*, ed. N. E. Robinson (Philadelphia: W. B. Saunders, 1992), 146–49.

14. A. J. Nixon, "Superficial Flexor Tendinitis," in *Current Practice of Equine Surgery*, 441.

15. R. L. Genovese et al., "Diagnostic Ultrasonography of Equine Limbs," *Vet. Clin. NA Eq. Prac.* 2, no. 1 (1986): 145–226.

16. R. Henninger, L. R. Bramlage and R. K. Schneider, "Short Term Effects of Superior Check Ligament Desmotomy and Percutaneous Tendon Splitting as a Treatment for Acute Tendinitis," *Proc. 36th AAEP* (1990): 539–40.

17. L. R. Bramlage, "Superior Check Ligament Desmotomy as a Treatment for Superficial Digital Flexor Tendinitis: Initial Report," *Proc. 32nd AAEP* (1986): 365–70.

CHAPTER FOURTEEN

1. W. Moyer, "Clinical Examination of the Equine Foot," *Vet. Clin. NA Eq. Prac.* 5, no. 1 (1989): 29.

2. T. A. Turner and C. Stork, "Hoof Abnormalities and Their Relation to Lameness," *Proc. 34th AAEP* (1988): 293–97.

3. O. Balch, K. White and D. Butler, "Factors Involved in the Balancing of Equine Hooves," *JAVMA* 198, no. 11 (1990): 1980–89.

4. O. Balch and S. Metcalf, *Farriery for Veterinarians* (Pullman, WA: S & O Press, 1990), 7, 8, 26, 34.

5. L. Emery, J. Miller and N. Van Hoosen, *Horseshoeing Theory and Hoof Care* (Philadelphia: Lea and Febiger, 1977), 72–75, 92, 100, 125.

6. C. Colles, "Interpreting Radiographs 1: The Foot," *Eq. Vet. J.*, 15 (1983): 297–303.

7. H. M. Clayton, "The Effect of an Acute Hoof Wall Angulation on the Stride Kinematics of Trotting Horses," *Eq. Vet. J.*, suppl. 9 (June 1990): 86–89.

8. H. M. Clayton, "Comparison of the Stride of Trotting Horses Trimmed with a Normal and Broken-Back Hoof Axis," *Proc. 33rd AAEP* (1987): 289–98.

9. O. K. Balch et al., "Locomotor Effect of Hoof Angle and Mediolateral Balance of Horses Exercising on a High-Speed Treadmill: Preliminary Results," *Proc. 37th AAEP* (1991): 687–705.

10. C. N. Kobluk et al., "The Effect of Conformation and Shoeing: A Cohort Study of 95 Thoroughbred Racehorses," *Proc. 35th AAEP* (1990): 259–74.

11. F. K. Lochner et al., "In Vivo and In Vitro Measurement of Tendon Strain in Horses," *Am. J. Vet. Res.* 41, no. 12 (1980): 1929–37.

12. K. N. Thompson, T. K. Cheung and M. Silverman, "The Effect of Toe Angle on Tendon, Ligament and Hoof Wall Strains in Vitro," *J. Eq. Vet. Sci.* 13, no. 11 (1993): 651–54.

13. K. Keegan et al., "Measurement of Suspensory Ligament Strain Using a Liquid Mercury Strain Gauge: Evaluation of Strain Reduction by Support Bandaging and Alteration of Hoof Wall Angle," *Proc. 37th AAEP* (1991): 243–44.

14. T. Bushe et al., "The Effect of Hoof Angle on Coffin, Pastern and Fetlock Joint Angles," *Proc. 33rd AAEP* (1987): 729–38.

15. W. Moyer, "Corrective Shoeing," *Vet. Clin. NA Large An. Prac.* 2, no. 1 (1980): 3–24.

16. R. A. Kainer, "Clinical Anatomy of the Equine Foot," *Vet. Clin. NA Eq. Prac.* 5, no. 1 (1989): 1–27.

17. L. J. Landeau, D. J. Barnett and S. C. Batterman, "Mechanical Properties of Equine Hooves," *Am. J. Vet. Res.* 44 (1983): 100.

18. S. A. Kempson, *Vet. Rec.* 120 (1987): 568.

19. N. Courben, R. J. Clark and D. J. B. Sutherland, *Vet. Rec.* 115 (1984): 642.

20. S. A. Kempson, "Ultrastructural Observation on the Response of Equine Hoof Defects to Dietary Supplementation with Farrier's Formula," *Vet. Rec.* 127 (1990): 494–98.

21. T. S. Stashak, *Adams' Lameness in Horses*, 4th ed. (Philadelphia: Lea and Febiger, 1987), 108–109.

22. M. J. Reeves, J. V. Yovich and A. S. Turner, "Miscellaneous Conditions of the Equine Foot," *Vet. Clin. NA Eq. Prac.* 5, no. 1 (1989): 235–36.

CHAPTER FIFTEEN

1. T. S. Stashak, *Adams' Lameness in Horses*, 4th ed. (Philadelphia: Lea and Febiger, 1987), 189.

2. M. A. Quddus, H. B. Kingsbury and J. R. Rooney, "A Force and Motion Study of the Foreleg of a Standardbred Trotter," *J. Eq. Med. Surg.* 2 (1978): 223–42.

3. G. W. Pratt, Jr., and J. T. O'Connor, Jr., "Force Plate Studies of Equine Biomechanics," *Am. J. Vet. Res.* 39 (1976): 249–53.

4. W. Moyer, "Clinical Examination of the Equine Foot," *Vet. Clin. NA Eq. Prac.* 5, no. 1 (1989): 29.

5. T. A. Turner and C. Stork, "Hoof Abnormalities and Their Relation to Lameness," *Proc. 34th AAEP* (1988): 293–97.

6. O. K. Balch et al., "Locomotor Effect of Hoof Angle and Mediolateral Balance of Horses Exercising on a High-Speed Treadmill: Preliminary Results," *Proc. 37th AAEP* (1991): 687–705.

7. R. A. Kainer, "Clinical Anatomy of the Equine Foot," *Vet. Clin. NA Eq. Prac.* 5, no. 1 (1989): 1–27.

8. Stashak, *Adams' Lameness*, 9–10.

9. R. R. Pool, D. M. Meagher and S. M. Stover, "Pathophysiology of Navicular Syndrome," *Vet. Clin. NA Eq. Prac.* 5, no. 1 (1989): 109–29.

10. T. A. Turner, "Navicular Disease," in *Current Practice of Equine Surgery*, ed. N. A. White and J. N. Moore (Philadelphia: J. B. Lippincott, 1990), 413–16.

11. T. A. Turner, "Diagnosis and Treatment of the Navicular Syndrome in Horses," *Vet. Clin. NA Eq. Prac.* 5, no. 1 (1989): 131–44.

12. T. A. Turner et al., "Radiographic Changes in the Navicular Bones of Normal Horses," *Proc. 32nd AAEP* (1987): 309–14.

13. B. Kaser-Hotz and G. Ueltschi, "Radiographic Appearance of the Navicular Bone in Sound Horses," *Vet. Radiol. and Ultrasound* 33, no. 1 (1992): 9–17.

14. N. Ackerman, "Radiographic Appearance of the Navicular Bone in Normal Horses, *Eq. Med. Rev.* 2, no. 5 (1992): 6.

15. D. R. Trout, W. J. Hornof and T. R. O'Brien, "Soft Tissue- and Bone-Phase Scintigraphy for Diagnosis of Navicular Disease in Horses," *JAVMA* 198, no. 1 (1991): 73–77.

16. R. R. Steckel, "The Role of Scintigraphy in the Lameness Evaluation," *Vet. Clin. NA Eq. Prac.* 7, no. 2 (1991): 207–38.

17. L. Ostblom, C. Lund and F. Melsen, "Navicular Bone Disease: Result of Treatment Using Egg-Bar Shoeing Technique," *Eq. Vet. J.* 16 (1984): 203.

18. W. Moyer, "Therapeutic Principles of Diseases of the Foot," *Proc. 27th AAEP* (1981): 453.

19. T. A. Turner, "Shoeing Principles for the Management of Navicular Disease," *JAVMA*, 189 (1986): 298.

20. R. J. Rose et al., "Studies on Isoxsuprine Hydrochloride for the Treatment of Navicular Disease," *Eq. Vet. J.* 15 (1983): 238.

21. A. S. Turner and C. M. Tucker, "The Evaluation of Isoxsuprine Hydrochloride for the Treatment of Navicular Disease: A Double Blind Study," *Eq. Vet. J.* 21, no. 5 (1989): 338–41.

22. T. A. Turner, "Management of Navicular Disease in Horses: An Update," *Mod. Vet. Prac.* 1 (1986): 24.

23. B. R. Jackman et al., "Palmar Digital Neurectomy in Horses, 57 Cases (1984–1990)," *Vet. Surg.* 22, no. 4 (1993): 285–88.

24. I. M. Wright, "Navicular Suspensory Desmotomy in the Treatment of Navicular Disease: Technique and Preliminary Results," *Eq. Vet. J.* 18 (1986): 443–46.

25. J. R. Field, "Equine Navicular Disease," *Vet. Comp. Orth. Traum.* 2 (1988): 108–10.

26. G. W. Trotter, "Therapy for Navicular Disease," *Comp. Cont. Ed.*, Sept. 1991: 1462–66.

CHAPTER SIXTEEN

1. B. V. Beaver, "Aggressive Behavior Problems," *Vet. Clin. NA Eq. Prac.* 2, no. 3 (1986): 635–44.

2. R. R. Keiper, "Social Structure," *Vet. Clin. NA Eq. Prac.* 2, no. 3 (1986): 465–84.

3. K. A. Houpt, "Stable Vices and Trailer Problems," *Vet. Clin. NA Eq. Prac.* 2, no. 3 (1986): 623–33.

4. N. H. Dodman et al., "Investigation into the Use of Narcotic Antagonists in the Treatment of a Stereotypic Behavior Pattern, [Crib-Biting] in the Horse," *Am. J. Vet. Res.* 48 (1987): 311–19.

5. E. Laggerweig et al., "The Twitch in Horses: A Variant of Acupuncture," *Science* 22 (1978): 1172–74.
6. J. G. Willard et al., "Effect of Diet on Cecal pH and Feed Behavior of Horses," *J. An. Sci.* 45 (1977): 87–93.
7. R. E. Salter and R. J. Hudson, "Habitat Utilization by Feral Horses in Western Alberta," *Naturaliste Can.* 105 (1978): 309–21.
8. V. L. Voith, "Principles of Learning," *Vet. Clin. NA Eq. Prac.* 2, no. 3 (1986): 485–506.
9. O. Pfungst, *Das Pferd des von Osten (Der Kluge Hans)* (Leipzig: Johannes Ambrosius Barth, 1907).

CHAPTER SEVENTEEN

1. T. S. Ford, "Obstruction and Rupture of the Urinary Tract," in *Current Therapy in Equine Medicine III*, ed. N. E. Robinson (Philadelphia: W. B. Saunders, 1992), 613–15.
2. I. K. M. Liu, "Ovarian Abnormalities," in *Current Therapy in Equine Medicine II*, ed. N. E. Robinson (Philadelphia: W. B. Saunders, 1987), 500–503.
3. T. S. Stashak, *Adams' Lameness in Horses*, 4th ed. (Philadelphia: Lea and Febiger, 1987), 130–33.
4. J. C. Harman, "Backs, Performance and Acupuncture," *Proc. 38th AAEP* (1992): 337–47.
5. A. M. Koterba, "Diagnosis and Management of the Normal and Abnormal Neonatal Foal: General Considerations," in *Equine Clinical Neonatology* (Philadelphia: Lea and Febiger, 1990), 3–6.
6. C. R. Sweeney, "Pleuropneumonia," in *Current Therapy II*, 592–96.
7. D. W. Scott, *Large Animal Dermatology* (Philadelphia: W. B. Saunders, 1988), 3.
8. S. B. Adams, C. H. Lanan and J. Masty, "Motility of the Distal Portion of the Jejunem and Pelvic Flexure in Ponies. Effects of Six Drugs," *Am. J. Vet. Res.* 45 (1984): 795–99.

Index

Acepromazine, side effects of, 42–43
Acupuncture, 28–29
Anemia, 9–10
Anesthetic nerve "blocks," 14
Antibiotics, 35–38; side effects of, 38
Anti-inflammatory drugs: non-steroidal, 40–42; steroidal, 38–40
Arthritis, 23, 143–46

Bandages: chronic inflammation and, 24; direction of, 21–22; granulation tissue and, 129; limb swelling and, 140–41; swelling and, 20–21; wound management and, 131–32
Bar shoes, 158
Blankets, 190
Blistering, 27–28
Bone scan. *See* Scintigraphy
Bots, 95
Botulism, 84–85
"Bowed" tendon, 147
Bran, 110, 111–12
"Breakover," of hoof, 155
Broken legs, 191–92
Bute. *See* Phenylbutazone

Canine teeth, 100
Chiropractic, 27–28
Choke, 59
Circulation, and healing, 25–26
Colic: and cribbing, 182; definition of, 105; and dehydration, 114; and diet, 110–11; and obesity, 62; prevention of, 110; and rolling, 109; signs of, 106; and walking the horse, 108–9; and the weather, 110

Colic surgery, 106–7
Communication, between horses, 184–85
Conformation, 141–42
Corn, 56
Counterirritants, 24
Creep feeding, 66
Cribbing, 59, 181–82
"Cystic" ovaries, 188

Dehydration and "skin pinch," 114–15
Dentists, 101
Deworming: compounds, 89–91; frequency of, 93; methods of administration, 91–92; nonchemical, 94; schedule, 92
Digestion, "hard" vs. "easy," 51
DMSO (dimethyl sulfoxide), 44–45
Dominance, 183–84
"Drawing out" abscesses, 29
Drugs, 33–34

Electrolytes, 61
Encephalitis, 82
Endotoxin, 85
Enemas, for foals, 189
Energy: of feeds, 50–51; supplementation for exercise, 55
Equine viral arteristis, 85
Exercise, and feeding, 55, 56, 57

Fat (feed supplement), 55
Fecal analysis, 94
Feed processing, 59
Feeding guidelines: adults, 54–55, 57–58, 64; foals, 66–67; during

gestation, 69–70; during lactation, 70; older horses, 70–71; up to two years, 69; weanlings, 68–69
Fever, 7–8
"Firing" limbs, 28
Flexion tests, 138–39
Flu. *See* Influenza
Foals, feeding of, 66–67
Founder. *See* Laminitis
Frog, importance of, 160–61

Grains, 55, 56–57
Granulation tissue, 127, 129–130
"Gravel," 162

Hair coat, growth of, 190
Hay, 52–53, 58–59; and the kidneys, 58–59; processed products, 59; requirements for, 54
Healing: delayed first intention, 128–29; first intention, 125–126; second intention, 127–28, 129
Heat: and inflammation, 13, 19; treatment for, 19–20
Hoof: abscesses, 162; angle, 152–53, 157–58; balance, 153; breakover, 160; flight, 154–55; growth of, 160; length, 153–54; supplements for, 161; testers, 14, 170; white vs. dark, 161
Hydrogen peroxide, 125

Illness, behavioral changes and, 4–6
Infection: vs. contamination, 126; vs. inflammation, 19
Inflammation: acute, 13, 19; chronic, 23–24
Influenza (flu), 78
Intelligence, 185
Isoxsuprine, 174–75

Kidneys: and alfalfa hay, 58–59; and back pain, 188

Lameness: physical examination and, 12–13; signs of, 137
Laminitis: grains and, 56–57; non-steroidal anti-inflammatory drugs and, 41; obesity and, 62; steroidal anti-inflammatory drugs and, 39
Learning, 185–87

Manure, eating of, 60–61
Milk, feeding and composition of, 70
Minerals, 52; abnormal eating and, 60–61; supplementation of in foals, 66–67
Mineral oil, 114, 189

Nails, in the foot, 136
Navicular bone, anatomy of, 165
Navicular disease: diagnosis of, 14, 169–73; heel soreness vs., 165–66; vs. "navicular syndrome," 166; prediction of, 171; "prenavicular," 169; prepurchase evaluations and, 171–72; signs of, 166–67; and stress tests, 170; surgery for, 175
Nerve "blocks," 14, 170–71
"Nerving" (neurectomy), 175
Non-steroidal anti-inflammatory drugs, 33, 40–42

Obesity, 54, 62
Orthopedic problems, developmental, 66–69
Ovaries, and back pain, 188

Pain, 22–23
Pain-relieving drugs, 22–23, 24
Parasites: and allergies, 89; and colic, 89, 112–13; and granulomas, 89; and pneumonia, 93; and weight loss, 88–89
Penicillin, and strangles, 119–21
Phenylbutazone, 33, 40
Potomac horse fever, 83–84

Poultices, 29
Protein, in feed, 51
"Proud cut" geldings, 192
Proud flesh. *See* Granulation tissue
Purpura hemorrhagica, 119
Putting to sleep, 192

Rabies, 84
Rectal examination, 8
Red blood cells, 9
Rhinopneumonitis, 78–80
Ringbone, 145–146

Sand, and colic, 113
Scar tissue: abdominals, 23; and ten-
    dons, 23; and wounds, 130–31
Scintigraphy, 16, 172
Serum chemistries, 11
Shipping horses, 189–90
Skin grafting, 131
Soaking feet, 29
Spavin, 143, 144
"Spooking," 179–80
Stall "vices," 59, 181–83
Steroidal anti-inflammatory drugs, 39,
    40
Stethoscope, 6
Stones, intestinal, 112
Strangles: complications of, 119; con-
    trol of, 117; development of, 116,
    and immunity, 121; internal
    abscesses and, 120–21; signs of,
    116–17; vaccination and, 86,
    118–19
Stride, length of versus toe length, 156
Support bandage, 140–41
"Sweat" wraps, 30
Swelling, limb, 20, 139

Teeth: and aging the horse, 100–101;
    and the bridle, 99–100; "floating"
    and, 97–98; frequency of examina-
tion and, 96–97; shedding of,
    98–99; of underweight horses,
    96–97, 98
Temperature, normal, 6
Tendon injuries, 146–50; and hoof
    angles, 156–57; rehabilitation of,
    149–50
Tendon sheath, 146
Tendon surgeries, 149
Tetanus, 80–82
Thermography, 13
Thrush, 163
Tranquilizers, 42–44
Tryptophane, 43–44
Twitch, mechanism of action, 182

Ultrasound, 15, 148
Underweight horse, 54, 62–63

Vaccinations: of foals, 189; frequency
    of, 76–78; and gestation, 79; killed
    vs. modified, 79; mechanism of
    action of, 76; reactions to, 86, 119;
    time off after, 86
Vinegar, and colic prevention, 112
Vitamins: and anemia, 10; and feeds,
    51; requirements for, 58–59

Water, 52, 64
Weaning, 68
Weanlings, feeding of, 68–69
White blood cells, function of, 10
Wild horses, 180–81
Wolf teeth, 100
Wood chewing, 182–83
Wound care: and bleeding, 124; and
    cleaning, 124; and dressings, 125,
    132; minor, 123
Wound infections, 126–27, 128
Wound repair, 125–31

X rays, 15, 137, 171–72